The American Psychiatric Association Practice Guideline for the Treatment of Patients With Eating Disorders

FOURTH EDITION

Guideline Writing Group

Catherine Crone, M.D., Chair
Laura J. Fochtmann, M.D., M.B.I.,
 Vice-Chair; Methodologist
Evelyn Attia, M.D.
Robert Boland, M.D.
Javier Escobar, M.D.
Victor Fornari, M.D., M.S.
Neville Golden, M.D.
Angela Guarda, M.D.
Maga Jackson-Triche, M.D., M.S.H.S.
Laurie Manzo, M.Ed., R.D., L.D.N.
Margherita Mascolo, M.D.
Karen Pierce, M.D.
Megan Riddle, M.D., Ph.D., M.S.
Andreea Seritan, M.D.
Blair Uniacke, M.D.
Nancy Zucker, Ph.D.

Systematic Review Group

Laura J. Fochtmann, M.D., M.B.I.,
 Methodologist
Joel Yager, M.D.
Thomas J. Craig, M.D.
Seung-Hee Hong
Jennifer Medicus

Committee on Practice Guidelines

Daniel J. Anzia, M.D., Chair
R. Scott Benson, M.D.
Catherine Crone, M.D.
Annette L. Hanson, M.D.
Michael J. Vergare, M.D.
Ilse Wiechers, M.D.
John M. Oldham, M.D.,
 Corresponding Member
Jacqueline Posada, M.D.,
 Corresponding Member
Joel Yager, M.D., Corresponding
 Member
Laura J. Fochtmann, M.D., M.B.I.,
 Medical Editor

APA Assembly Liaisons

Daniel Dahl, M.D.
Evan Eyler, M.D.
Jason W. Hunziker, M.D.
Marvin Koss, M.D.
Lisa Schock, M.D.

APA and the Guideline Writing Group especially thank Laura J. Fochtmann, M.D., M.B.I., Blair Uniacke, M.D., Seung-Hee Hong, and Jennifer Medicus for their outstanding work and effort in developing this guideline. APA also wishes to acknowledge the contributions of other APA staff including Michelle Dirst, Andrew Lyzenga, and Kristin Kroeger Ptakowski. APA wishes to give special recognition to Joel Yager, M.D. for his decades of contributions to APA and its practice guidelines, including his work on the Systematic Review Group and serving as Chair of the Eating Disorders Writing Group for three prior versions of this guideline. APA also thanks the APA Committee on Practice Guidelines (Daniel J. Anzia, M.D., Chair), liaisons from the APA Assembly for their input and assistance, and APA Councils and others for providing feedback during the comment period.

For inquiries about permissions or licensing, please contact Permissions & Licensing, American Psychiatric Association Publishing, 800 Maine Avenue SW, Suite 900, Washington, DC 20024-2812 or submit inquiries online at: www.appi.org/Support/Customer-Information/Permissions.

If you wish to buy 50 or more copies of the same title, please go to www.appi.org/specialdiscounts for more information.

Copyright © 2023 American Psychiatric Association

ISBN 978-0-89042-584-8

ALL RIGHTS RESERVED

Fourth Edition

Manufactured in the United States of America on acid-free paper
27 26 25 24 23   5 4 3 2 1

American Psychiatric Association
800 Maine Avenue SW, Suite 900
Washington, DC 20024-2812
www.appi.org

Library of Congress Cataloging-in-Publication Data
A CIP record is available from the Library of Congress.

British Library Cataloguing in Publication Data
A CIP record is available from the British Library.

Contents

Acronyms/Abbreviations

AACAP   American Academy of Child and Adolescent Psychiatry

AAP   American Academy of Pediatrics

ACOG   American College of Obstetricians and Gynecologists

ADHD   attention-deficit/hyperactivity disorder

AFT   adolescent-focused therapy

AHRQ   Agency for Healthcare Research and Quality

AN   anorexia nervosa

APA   American Psychiatric Association

ARFID   avoidant/restrictive food intake disorder

BDI   Beck Depression Inventory

BED   binge-eating disorder

BES   Binge Eating Scale

BMD   bone mineral density

BMI   body mass index

BN   bulimia nervosa

BWL   behavioral weight loss

CBT   cognitive-behavioral therapy

CBT-E   enhanced cognitive-behavioral therapy

CGI   Clinical Global Impression

CI   confidence interval; credible interval (when used in describing network meta-analysis results)

CPT   Current Procedural Terminology

CRT   cognitive remediation therapy

DBT   dialectical behavior therapy

DHEA   dehydroepiandrosterone

DIC   deviation information criterion

DSM   *Diagnostic and Statistical Manual of Mental Disorders*

DSM-IV   *Diagnostic and Statistical Manual of Mental Disorders*, 4th Edition

DSM-5   *Diagnostic and Statistical Manual of Mental Disorders*, 5th Edition

DXA   dual X-ray absorptiometry

EBW   expected body weight

ECG   electrocardiogram

ECHO   Experienced Caregivers Helping Others

ECT   electroconvulsive therapy

EDE   Eating Disorder Examination

EDE-Q   Eating Disorder Examination Questionnaire

EE   expressed emotion

EHR   electronic health record

ERP   exposure and response prevention

FBT   family-based treatment/therapy

FPT   focal psychodynamic psychotherapy

GFR   glomerular filtration rate

GI   gastrointestinal

GRADE   Grading of Recommendations Assessment, Development and Evaluation

GSH   guided self-help

GWG   Guideline Writing Group

IBW   ideal body weight

IPT   interpersonal psychotherapy

MANTRA   Maudsley Model of Anorexia Nervosa Treatment for Adults

MET   motivational enhancement therapy

NESARC-III   National Epidemiologic Survey Alcohol and Related Conditions–III

NGT   nasogastric tube

NIMH   National Institute of Mental Health

NMA   network meta-analysis

OCD   obsessive-compulsive disorder

OR   odds ratio

OTC   over-the-counter

PARDI   Pica, ARFID, and Rumination Disorder Interview

PTSD   posttraumatic stress disorder

RCT   randomized controlled trial

RDoC   Research Domain Criteria

RMD   relative mean difference

RR   relative risk

SD   standard deviation

SEM   standard error of the mean

SPT   supportive psychotherapy

SRG   Systematic Review Group

SSCM   Specialist Supportive Clinical Management

SSRI   selective serotonin reuptake inhibitor

TAU   treatment as usual

Introduction

Rationale

The goal of this guideline is to improve the quality of care and treatment outcomes for patients with eating disorders, as defined by the *Diagnostic and Statistical Manual of Mental Disorders*, 5th Edition (DSM-5; American Psychiatric Association 2013). As described in "Scope of Document," we focus primarily on anorexia nervosa (AN), bulimia nervosa (BN), and binge-eating disorder (BED) rather than other DSM-defined feeding and eating disorders. Since publication of the last American Psychiatric Association (APA) practice guideline (American Psychiatric Association 2006) and guideline watch on eating disorders (Yager et al. 2012), there have been many studies on psychotherapies for individuals with these diagnoses as well as some studies on pharmacotherapies. Despite this, there are still substantial gaps in the availability and use of evidence-based treatments for individuals with an eating disorder (Kazdin et al. 2017). This practice guideline aims to help clinicians improve care for their patients by reviewing current evidence and providing evidence-based statements that are intended to enhance knowledge, increase assessment, and optimize treatment of eating disorders.

The lifetime prevalence of eating disorders in the United States is approximately 0.80% for AN, 0.28% for BN, and 0.85% for BED (Udo and Grilo 2018), although estimates can vary depending on the study location, sample demographic characteristics, case finding, and diagnostic approaches (Galmiche et al. 2019; Santomauro et al. 2021; Wu et al. 2020). For example, the prevalence of an eating disorder appears to be higher in LGBTQ+ individuals than in cisgender heterosexual peers (Kamody et al. 2020; Nagata et al. 2020b). Furthermore, data suggest an increasing incidence of eating disorders and inpatient care for eating disorders, particularly AN, during the COVID-19 pandemic (Agostino et al. 2021; Asch et al. 2021; Otto et al. 2021; Taquet et al. 2021). Importantly, the lifetime burdens and psychosocial impairments associated with an eating disorder can be substantial because these illnesses can persist for decades, and they typically have an onset in adolescence or early adulthood (Udo and Grilo 2018).

In the United States, for the 2018–2019 fiscal year, the total economic costs of eating disorders were estimated to be $64.7 billion, with an additional $326.5 billion attributable to reductions in well-being associated with eating disorders (Streatfeild et al. 2021). Of total economic costs, AN represented 17% of costs, BN 18% of costs, and BED 30% of costs (Streatfeild et al. 2021). Evidence from other countries is consistent with the United States' findings and emphasizes the high economic burdens associated with eating disorders (Jenkins 2022; Tannous et al. 2021; van Hoeken and Hoek 2020).

Eating disorders are associated with increases in all-cause mortality and in deaths due to suicide (Auger et al. 2021; Nielsen and Vilmar 2021; Tith et al. 2020; van Hoeken and Hoek 2020). With AN, the increases in risks of mortality and premature death are substantially greater in men than in women (Edakubo and Fushimi 2020; Fichter et al. 2021; Iwajomo et al. 2021; Quadflieg et al. 2019), although the absolute numbers of deaths associated with an eating disorder are greater in women. Rates of suicide attempts are also increased in individuals who have an eating disorder (Keski-Rahkonen 2021; Smith et al. 2018; Udo et al. 2019). Morbidity and mortality among individuals with an eating disorder are heightened by the common co-occurrence of health conditions, such as diabetes, and of other psychiatric disorders, particularly depression, anxiety, posttraumatic stress disorder (PTSD), obsessive-compulsive disorder (OCD), attention-deficit/hyperactivity disorder (ADHD),

1

and substance use disorders (Ahn et al. 2019; Cliffe et al. 2020; Gibbings et al. 2021; Keski-Rahkonen 2021; Udo and Grilo 2019).

Accordingly, the overall goal of this guideline is to enhance the assessment and treatment of eating disorders, thereby reducing the mortality, morbidity, and significant psychosocial and health consequences of these important psychiatric conditions.

Scope of Document

This practice guideline focuses on evidence-based pharmacological, psychotherapeutic, and other nonpharmacological treatments for eating disorders in adolescents, emerging adults, and adults. In addition, it includes statements related to assessment and treatment planning, which are an integral part of patient-centered care.

The scope of this document is shaped by the diagnostic criteria for eating disorders and by the available evidence as obtained by a systematic review of the literature through September 2021. In particular, it focuses on AN, BN, and BED as defined by DSM-III, DSM-III-R, DSM-IV, DSM-IV-TR, DSM-5, or ICD-10. Some of the studies included individuals whose symptoms were below the threshold for a diagnosis of AN, BN, or BED, but these data were rarely analyzed separately in a way that would permit unique recommendations to be crafted for this group of patients. Nevertheless, some guideline statements may also be relevant to individuals with unspecified or other specified feeding or eating disorders.

Our systematic review attempted to include literature on avoidant/restrictive food intake disorder (ARFID); however, rigorous clinical trial data were not available due to the relative recency of the introduction of this diagnosis. Consequently, none of the guideline statements are related to the treatment of ARFID. However, we have included some discussion of ARFID in the implementation sections of this document, particularly as it relates to assessment and treatment planning.

We specifically excluded rumination disorder and pica from our search of the literature due to their typical age of onset in infancy or childhood and the limited evidence on their treatment. We also excluded treatment of obesity from the scope of this guideline because obesity is not categorized as an eating disorder. Although obesity is common among individuals who are treated in psychiatric practice, literature on obesity is already summarized by practice guidelines from other organizations and professional societies.

Most studies reported including a preponderance of women, typically adolescents or young adults, but participants' genders were not described more fully. Most studies also enrolled predominantly white participants or did not specify the racial, ethnic, or cultural characteristics of the sample. These limitations of the evidence should be considered in terms of the document scope and the compelling need for additional research in more representative samples. In addition, as evidence accrues and as social norms change, terminology will likely evolve as well (Flanagin et al. 2021; OHSU Center for Diversity and Inclusion 2021).

Data are also limited on individuals with eating disorders and significant physical health conditions or co-occurring psychiatric conditions, including substance use disorders. Many of the available studies of eating disorders did not analyze data separately for these patient subgroups or excluded individuals with these comorbidities. Nevertheless, in the absence of more robust evidence, the statements in this guideline should generally be applicable to individuals with co-occurring conditions.

Our systematic review did not include studies for preventive interventions (Harrer et al. 2020; Stice et al. 2021; Watson et al. 2016) or risk factors for eating disorders, such as frequent dieting behaviors, childhood abuse, or bullying (Emery et al. 2021; Hooper et al. 2021; Lie et al. 2019; Solmi et al. 2021; Yoon et al. 2020). It also did not include search terms to identify literature on stigma and discrimination, either as risk factors for eating disorders, contributors to symptoms, or barriers to seeking treatment (Ali et al. 2017; Brelet et al. 2021; Bristow et al. 2020; Foran et al. 2020; Hamilton et al. 2022; O'Connor et al. 2021). Each of these topics is important but would warrant a distinct systematic review from one focused on treatments for eating disorders. Cost-effectiveness considerations are also outside of the scope of this guideline. Although treatment-related costs are often barriers to receiving treatment, costs of treatment typically differ by country and geographical region and vary widely by health system and payment model. In addition, few high-quality studies exist on the cost-effectiveness of treatments for eating disorders that could be used to inform health care policy.

Although we discuss studies of specific psychotherapies that were delivered via a Web-based approach, we do not discuss telehealth as a specific intervention because there were no direct comparisons of telehealth and in-person care prior to 2020. The rapidly expanding literature on the use of telehealth (Anderson et al. 2017; Blalock et al. 2020; Levinson et al. 2021; Matheson et al. 2020; Raykos et al. 2021; Stewart et al. 2021; Waller et al. 2020), Web-based interventions (Barakat et al. 2019), and mobile applications (Anastasiadou et al. 2018; Linardon et al. 2020; Wasil et al. 2021) in the treatment of eating disorders will help to inform future practice guidelines.

Overview of the Development Process

Since the publication of *Clinical Practice Guidelines We Can Trust* (Institute of Medicine 2011a), a report of the Institute of Medicine (now known as National Academy of Medicine), there has been an increasing focus on using clearly defined, transparent processes for rating the quality of evidence and the strength of the overall body of evidence in systematic reviews of the scientific literature. This guideline was developed using a process intended to be consistent with the recommendations of the Institute of Medicine (2011a) and *Principles for the Development of Specialty Society Clinical Guidelines* of the Council of Medical Specialty Societies (2012). The parameters used for the guideline's systematic review are included with the full text of the guideline; the development process is fully described in the following document, which is available at the APA website: www.psychiatry.org/ psychiatrists/practice/clinical-practice-guidelines/guideline-development-process.

Rating the Strengths of Guideline Statements and Supporting Research Evidence

Development of guideline statements entails weighing the potential benefits and harms of the statement and then identifying the level of confidence in that determination. (See Appendix G for detailed descriptions of the potential benefits and harms for each statement.) This concept of balancing benefits and harms to determine guideline recommendations and strength of recommendations is a hallmark of GRADE (Grading of Recommendations Assessment, Development and Evaluation), which is used by multiple professional organizations around the world to develop practice guideline recommendations (Guyatt et al. 2013). With the GRADE approach, recommendations are rated by assessing the confidence that the benefits of the statement outweigh the harms and burdens of the statement, determining the confidence in estimates of effect as reflected by the quality of evidence, estimating patient values and preferences (including whether they are similar across the patient population), and identifying whether resource expenditures are worth the expected net benefit of following the recommendation (Andrews et al. 2013).

In weighing the balance of benefits and harms for each statement in this guideline, our level of confidence is informed by available evidence (see Appendix C), which includes evidence from clinical trials as well as expert opinion and patient values and preferences. Evidence for the benefit of a particular intervention within a specific clinical context is identified through systematic review and is then balanced against the evidence for harms. In this regard, harms are broadly defined and may include serious adverse events, less serious adverse events that affect tolerability, minor adverse events, negative effects of the intervention on quality of life, barriers and inconveniences associated with treatment, direct and indirect costs of the intervention (including opportunity costs), and other negative aspects of the treatment that may influence decision-making by the patient, the clinician, or both.

Many topics covered in this guideline have relied on forms of evidence such as consensus opinions of experienced clinicians or indirect findings from observational studies rather than research from randomized trials. It is well recognized that there are guideline topics and clinical circumstances for which high-quality evidence from clinical trials is not possible or is unethical to obtain (Council of Medical Specialty Societies 2012). For example, many questions need to be asked as part of an assessment, and inquiring about a particular symptom or element of the history cannot be separated out for study as a discrete intervention. It would also be impossible to separate changes in outcomes due to assessment from changes in outcomes due to ensuing treatment. Research on psychiatric assessments and some psychiatric interventions can also be complicated by multiple confounding factors such as the interaction between the clinician and the patient or the patient's unique circumstances and experiences. The GRADE working group and guidelines developed by other professional organizations have noted that a strong recommendation or "good practice statement" may be appropriate even in the absence of research evidence when sensible alternatives do not exist (Andrews et al. 2013; Brito et al. 2013; Djulbegovic et al. 2009; Hazlehurst et al. 2013). For each guideline statement, we have described the type and strength of the available evidence as well as the factors, including patient preferences, that were used in determining the balance of benefits and harms.

The authors of the guideline determined each final rating, as described in the section "Guideline Development Process" (see Table 1). A *recommendation* (denoted by the numeral 1 after the guideline statement) indicates confidence that the benefits of the intervention clearly outweigh harms. A *suggestion* (denoted by the numeral 2 after the guideline statement) indicates greater uncertainty. Although the benefits of the statement are still viewed as outweighing the harms, the balance of benefits and harms is more difficult to judge, or either the benefits or the harms may be less clear. With a suggestion, patient values and preferences may be more variable, and this can influence the clinical decision that is ultimately made. Each guideline statement also has an associated rating for the *strength of supporting research evidence*. Three ratings are used: *high, moderate,* and *low* (denoted by the letters A, B, and C, respectively) and reflect the level of confidence that the evidence for a guideline statement reflects a true effect based on consistency of findings across studies, directness of the effect on a specific health outcome, precision of the estimate of effect, and risk of bias in available studies (Agency for Healthcare Research and Quality 2014; Balshem et al. 2011; Guyatt et al. 2006).

TABLE 1. Rating the strengths of guideline statements and evidence for guideline statements

Strength of guideline statement			Strength of evidence		
1	Recommendation	Denotes confidence that the benefits of the intervention clearly outweigh the harms.	A	High confidence	Further research is very unlikely to change the estimate of effect and our confidence in it.
2	Suggestion	Denotes benefits that are viewed as outweighing harms, but the balance is more difficult to judge and patient values and preferences may be more variable.	B	Moderate confidence	Further research may change the estimate of effect and our confidence in it.
			C	Low confidence	Further research is likely to change the estimate of effect and our confidence in it.

Proper Use of Guidelines

The APA Practice Guidelines are assessments of current (as of the date of authorship) scientific and clinical information provided as an educational service. The guidelines 1) should not be considered as a statement of the standard of care or inclusive of all proper treatments or methods of care; 2) are not continually updated and may not reflect the most recent evidence, as new evidence may emerge between the time information is developed and when the guidelines are published or read; 3) address only the question(s) or issue(s) specifically identified; 4) do not mandate any particular course of medical care; 5) are not intended to substitute for the independent professional judgment of the treating clinician; and 6) do not account for individual variation among patients. As such, it is not possible to draw conclusions about the effects of omitting a particular recommendation, either in general or for a specific patient. Furthermore, adherence to these guidelines will not ensure a successful outcome for every individual, nor should these guidelines be interpreted as including all proper methods of evaluation and care or excluding other acceptable methods of evaluation and care aimed at the same results. The ultimate recommendation regarding a particular assessment, clinical procedure, or treatment plan must be made by the clinician directly involved in the patient's care in light of the psychiatric evaluation, other clinical data, and the diagnostic and treatment options available. Such recommendations should be made in collaboration with the patient whenever possible and should incorporate the patient's personal and sociocultural preferences and values, which can enhance the therapeutic alliance, adherence to treatment, and treatment outcomes. For all of these reasons, the APA cautions against the use of guidelines in litigation. Use of these guidelines is voluntary. APA provides the guidelines on an "as is" basis and makes no warranty, expressed or implied, regarding them. APA assumes no responsibility for any injury or damage to persons or property arising out of or related to any use of the guidelines or for any errors or omissions.

A Note About This Guideline

For ease of clinical use, only the guideline statements and the discussion of their implementation are included in the print version. Discussion of the research evidence and a detailed description of the guideline development process are available online at https://psychiatryonline.org/doi/book/10.1176/appi.books.9780890424865.

Guideline Statement Summary

Assessment and Determination of Treatment Plan

1. APA *recommends* **(1C)** screening for the presence of an eating disorder as part of an initial psychiatric evaluation.
2. APA *recommends* **(1C)** that the initial evaluation of a patient with a possible eating disorder include assessment of

   - the patient's height and weight history (e.g., maximum and minimum weight, recent weight changes);
   - presence of, patterns in, and changes in restrictive eating, food avoidance, binge eating, and other eating-related behaviors (e.g., rumination, regurgitation, chewing and spitting);
   - patterns and changes in food repertoire (e.g., breadth of food variety, narrowing or elimination of food groups);
   - presence of, patterns in, and changes in compensatory and other weight control behaviors, including dietary restriction, compulsive or driven exercise, purging behaviors (e.g., laxative use, self-induced vomiting), and use of medication to manipulate weight;
   - percentage of time preoccupied with food, weight, and body shape;
   - prior treatment and response to treatment for an eating disorder;
   - psychosocial impairment secondary to eating or body image concerns or behaviors; and
   - family history of eating disorders, other psychiatric illnesses, and other medical conditions (e.g., obesity, inflammatory bowel disease, diabetes mellitus).

3. APA *recommends* **(1C)** that the initial psychiatric evaluation of a patient with a possible eating disorder include weighing the patient and quantifying eating and weight control behaviors (e.g., frequency, intensity, or time spent on dietary restriction, binge eating, purging, exercise, and other compensatory behaviors).
4. APA *recommends* **(1C)** that the initial psychiatric evaluation of a patient with a possible eating disorder identify co-occurring health conditions, including co-occurring psychiatric disorders.
5. APA *recommends* **(1C)** that the initial psychiatric evaluation of a patient with a possible eating disorder include a comprehensive review of systems.
6. APA *recommends* **(1C)** that the initial physical examination of a patient with a possible eating disorder include assessment of vital signs, including temperature, resting heart rate, blood pressure, orthostatic pulse, and orthostatic blood pressure; height, weight, and body mass index (BMI; or percent median BMI, BMI percentile, or BMI Z-score for children and adolescents); and physical appearance, including signs of malnutrition or purging behaviors.
7. APA *recommends* **(1C)** that the laboratory assessment of a patient with a possible eating disorder include a complete blood count and a comprehensive metabolic panel, including electrolytes, liver enzymes, and renal function tests.
8. APA *recommends* **(1C)** that an electrocardiogram be done in patients with a restrictive eating disorder, patients with severe purging behavior, and patients who are taking medications that are known to prolong QTc intervals.
9. APA *recommends* **(1C)** that patients with an eating disorder have a documented, comprehensive, culturally appropriate, and person-centered treatment plan that incorporates medical, psychiatric, psychological, and nutritional expertise, commonly via a coordinated multidisciplinary team.

Anorexia Nervosa

10. APA *recommends* **(1C)** that patients with anorexia nervosa who require nutritional rehabilitation and weight restoration have individualized goals set for weekly weight gain and target weight.
11. APA *recommends* **(1B)** that adults with anorexia nervosa be treated with an eating disorder–focused psychotherapy, which should include normalizing eating and weight control behaviors, restoring weight, and addressing psychological aspects of the disorder (e.g., fear of weight gain, body image disturbance).
12. APA *recommends* **(1B)** that adolescents and emerging adults with anorexia nervosa who have an involved caregiver be treated with eating disorder–focused family-based treatment, which should include caregiver education aimed at normalizing eating and weight control behaviors and restoring weight.

Bulimia Nervosa

13. APA *recommends* **(1C)** that adults with bulimia nervosa be treated with eating disorder–focused cognitive-behavioral therapy and that a serotonin reuptake inhibitor (e.g., 60 mg fluoxetine daily) also be prescribed, either initially or if there is minimal or no response to psychotherapy alone by 6 weeks of treatment.
14. APA *suggests* **(2C)** that adolescents and emerging adults with bulimia nervosa who have an involved caregiver be treated with eating disorder–focused family-based treatment.

Binge-Eating Disorder

15. APA *recommends* **(1C)** that patients with binge-eating disorder be treated with eating disorder–focused cognitive-behavioral therapy or interpersonal therapy, in either individual or group formats.
16. APA *suggests* **(2C)** that adults with binge-eating disorder who prefer medication or have not responded to psychotherapy alone be treated with either an antidepressant medication or lisdexamfetamine.

Guideline Statements and Implementation

Assessment and Determination of Treatment Plan

STATEMENT 1: Screening for Presence of an Eating Disorder

APA *recommends* (1C) screening for the presence of an eating disorder as part of an initial psychiatric evaluation.

Implementation

Estimates of the prevalence and disease burden associated with eating disorders vary by country and depend on the methodology of the epidemiological study (Galmiche et al. 2019; Santomauro et al. 2021; Wu et al. 2020). Among individuals in the United States assessed in the 2012–2013 National Epidemiologic Survey Alcohol and Related Conditions-III (NESARC-III), the 12-month prevalence estimates for AN, BN, and BED were 0.05% (standard error of the mean [SEM] 0.02%), 0.14% (SEM 0.02%), and 0.44% (SEM 0.04%), whereas lifetime estimates were 0.80% (SEM 0.07%), 0.28% (SEM 0.03%), and 0.85% (SEM 0.05%), respectively (Udo and Grilo 2018). Somewhat different estimates were found in prior smaller studies such as the National Comorbidity Replication Survey (Hudson et al. 2007) and pooled data from the National Institute of Mental Health (NIMH) Collaborative Psychiatric Epidemiological Studies (Marques et al. 2011). Other studies suggest that the prevalence of eating disorders may be increasing (Favaro et al. 2009; Galmiche et al. 2019). Furthermore, many of these studies did not fully assess for unspecified or other specified eating disorders. As a result, the actual burden of eating disorders is likely to be underestimated (Feltner et al. 2021; Harrop et al. 2021; U.S. Preventive Services Task Force 2022; Ward et al. 2019).

In the NESARC-III findings, women were more likely to have a 12-month diagnosis or a lifetime diagnosis as compared to men (adjusted odds ratio [OR] for 12-month diagnosis 6.48 for AN, 5.16 for BN, and 2.37 for BED, and for lifetime diagnosis 12.00 for AN, 5.80 for BN, and 3.01 for BED; Udo and Grilo 2018). A lifetime diagnosis of BN was just as likely in Hispanic white and non-Hispanic Black individuals as in non-Hispanic white individuals; however, a lifetime diagnosis of AN was more likely in non-Hispanic white individuals than in Hispanic and non-Hispanic Black individuals, whereas BED was more common in non-Hispanic white than non-Hispanic Black individuals (Udo and Grilo 2018). LGBTQ+ individuals were also more likely to have a lifetime eating disorder diagnosis than cisgender heterosexual individuals, with adjusted ORs of 1.93 for AN, 3.69 for BN, 2.32 for BED, and 1.96 for any eating disorder (Kamody et al. 2020). In addition, more recent data suggest an increasing incidence of eating disorders and inpatient care for eating disorders, particularly AN, during the COVID-19 pandemic, and these increases appear to be unrelated to prior COVID-19 infection (Agostino et al. 2021; Asch et al. 2021; Lin et al. 2021; Otto et al. 2021; Taquet et al. 2021; Toulany et al. 2022).

The U.S. Preventive Services Task Force (2022) notes that there is insufficient evidence for routine screening for eating disorders in adolescents and adults (age 10 years or older) who have no signs or symptoms of an eating disorder. On the other hand, it can be challenging to identify eating disorder signs, symptoms, or risk factors without specific attention to these elements during the evaluation.

In addition, it is important to note that the presence of an eating disorder diagnosis cannot be predicted simply by assessing weight or BMI. Data from the Collaborative Psychiatric Epidemiology Surveys of 2001–2003 showed an increase in the adjusted OR for any 12-month or lifetime eating disorder among overweight and obese men and women relative to normal-weight individuals, with the greatest increase among those with Class III obesity (Duncan et al. 2017). Women with a low BMI also had an increased adjusted OR of any 12-month or lifetime eating disorder, but most underweight adults did not meet criteria for an eating disorder (Duncan et al. 2017). Furthermore, many individuals with an eating disorder do not receive help, even when this is broadly defined to include use of self-help or support groups. In the NESARC-III study, the prevalence of seeking any help was 34.5% for AN, 34.5% for BN, and 62.6% for BED, but there was substantial variability based on sex, race, and ethnicity (Coffino et al. 2019). In AN, the likelihood of seeking help was less in Hispanic as compared to non-Hispanic white individuals (adjusted OR 0.30), whereas in BED the likelihood of seeking help was less in men than in women (adjusted OR 0.29) and in non-Hispanic Black individuals (adjusted OR 0.25) and Hispanic individuals (adjusted OR 0.46) as compared to non-Hispanic white individuals (Coffino et al. 2019). Consequently, screening for eating disorder symptoms will be important in order to identify eating disorders and to reduce disparities in receipt of treatment (Marques et al. 2011). Systematically collected prevalence data are less available in gender-diverse individuals, but there appear to be higher rates of eating disorder diagnoses as well as weight and shape concerns among transgender and gender non-binary youth as compared to cisgender youth (Coelho et al. 2019; Grammer et al. 2021). Early recognition of an eating disorder is also essential because of the relatively young age of onset for eating disorders in many individuals. More specifically, the median age of onset in the NESARC-III study was 17.4 years in AN, 16.0 years in BN, and 21.1 years in BED (Udo and Grilo 2018), although some studies suggest that the median age of onset has been decreasing in recent years (Favaro et al. 2009; Galmiche et al. 2019). Mean ages of onset were slightly higher (Udo and Grilo 2018). A long duration of illness was common in the NESARC-III study, with a median duration of the episode of illness of 4.9 years in AN, 8.0 years in BN, and 10.6 years in BED; mean episode durations were 11.4 years (SEM 0.4), 12.2 years (SEM 0.67), and 15.9 years (SEM 0.36), respectively (Udo and Grilo 2018). Psychosocial impairment was also common in individuals with an eating disorder, highlighting the importance of early identification and intervention (Udo and Grilo 2018). For example, in individuals with AN, onset before 15 years of age was associated with greater illness severity, higher rates of lifetime psychiatric comorbidity, and more psychosocial difficulties (Grilo and Udo 2021).

Given the prevalence and typical age of onset of eating disorders in adolescence or young adulthood, the American Academy of Pediatrics recommends that pediatricians ask all preteens and adolescents about eating patterns and body image as well as screen for eating disorders and be alert to potential signs and symptoms of disordered eating (Hornberger et al. 2021).

Prevalence rates of eating disorders among patients receiving psychiatric treatment are likely to be considerably higher than in the general population, given the significant co-occurrence of eating disorders with other psychiatric disorders (see Statement 4). For example, one study of 260 individuals referred to a community-based mental health service for treatment of anxiety or depression noted ratings of eating problems (as measured by a score above 1 on the SCOFF) in 18.5% and a DSM-IV (American Psychiatric Association 1994) eating disorder in 7.3% of the total sample (Fursland and Watson 2014).

Other individuals who appear to have an increased likelihood of an eating disorder include individuals who have experienced teasing or bullying (Day et al. 2022; Lie et al. 2019; Solmi et al. 2021) or childhood sexual abuse (Solmi et al. 2021), athletes (Eichstadt et al. 2020; Sundgot-Borgen and Torstveit 2004), and patients with celiac disease (Lebwohl et al. 2021; Mårild et al. 2017) or type 1 diabetes mellitus (Hall et al. 2021; Toni et al. 2017). Despite their prevalence and importance, eating disorders may remain undetected unless systematic screening occurs. Individuals with an eating disorder may not have insight into the presence or severity of eating disorder signs and symptoms (Arbel et al. 2014; Gorwood et al. 2019; Konstantakopoulos et al. 2011, 2020). Males and individuals from racial, ethnic, and gender minorities may be less likely to be asked about the presence of eating disorder symptoms due to a perception that eating disorders primarily affect certain demographic groups (e.g., young white females). However, eating disorders occur among all populations, age groups, genders, and cultural groups, although clinical presentations may vary (Alegria et al. 2007; Cachelin and Striegel-Moore 2006; Hudson et al. 2007; Makino et al. 2004; Marques et al. 2011; Ricciardelli et al. 2007; Taylor et al. 2007; Udo and Grilo 2018). In fact, eating disorder diagnoses may be more frequent among transgender and gender non-binary individuals than in those who identify as cisgender (Coelho et al. 2019; Grammer et al. 2021). Clinicians may also erroneously overlook an eating disorder, including atypical AN, in individuals whose BMI is in the normal range or higher. To this end, the clinician should be sure to ask all patients about the presence of eating disorder symptoms as part of their standard psychiatric evaluation. For example, as part of the clinical interview, a patient could be asked "Have you or others worried that your preoccupation with weight, body shape, or food is excessive?" and "Have you felt that your weight or body shape excessively affects how you feel about yourself?" Screening questionnaires can also be used (see Table 2), although questions may need to be adapted based on the patient's developmental and cognitive level. In terms of structured rating scales, the SCOFF questionnaire is most frequently used for screening purposes (Kutz et al. 2020; Morgan et al. 1999). It is a five-item tool that has been translated into multiple languages (e.g., Garcia et al. 2010; Garcia-Campayo et al. 2005; Richter et al. 2017), has been studied in adolescents as well as adults (Kutz et al. 2020), and can be used as a written self-report tool or with questions asked by the interviewer (Perry et al. 2002). The SCOFF has high sensitivity and specificity (Morgan et al. 1999), particularly for identifying the presence of AN or BN in young women with eating disorder symptoms who have two or more positive responses to the SCOFF questions (Kutz et al. 2020). In more diverse populations, the predictive value of the SCOFF is reduced (Kutz et al. 2020; Solmi et al. 2015). It may also have less ability to detect unspecified or other specified feeding or eating disorders, including atypical AN (Maguen et al. 2018). In addition, it was developed before criteria for BED were established, and it performs less well in detecting the presence of BED (Kutz et al. 2020). For this reason, the SCOFF could be supplemented by adding the initial question from Binge Eating Disorder Screener–7 (Herman et al. 2016): "During the last 3 months, did you have any episodes of excessive overeating (i.e., eating significantly more than what most people would eat in a similar period of time)?" A follow-up question could ask whether any such episodes were associated with a loss of control or inability to stop eating.

Other questionnaires, including the Screen for Disordered Eating (Maguen et al. 2018) and the Eating Disorder Screen for Primary Care (Cotton et al. 2003), have also been proposed as screening tools. Both have a greater sensitivity than the SCOFF (Cotton et al. 2003; Maguen et al. 2018), but these screening tools have not been well studied among representative patient populations.

STATEMENT 2: Initial Evaluation of Eating History

APA *recommends* (1C) that the initial evaluation of a patient with a possible eating disorder include assessment of

- the patient's height and weight history (e.g., maximum and minimum weight, recent weight changes);
- presence of, patterns in, and changes in restrictive eating, food avoidance, binge eating, and other eating-related behaviors (e.g., rumination, regurgitation, chewing and spitting);
- patterns and changes in food repertoire (e.g., breadth of food variety, narrowing or elimination of food groups);
- presence of, patterns in, and changes in compensatory and other weight control behaviors, including dietary restriction, compulsive or driven exercise, purging behaviors (e.g., laxative use, self-induced vomiting), and use of medication to manipulate weight;

TABLE 2. Screening questionnaires for eating disorders

SCOFF Questionnaire (Morgan et al. 1999)

Do you make yourself **S**ick because you feel uncomfortably full?

Do you worry you have lost **C**ontrol over how much you eat?

Have you recently lost >14 lbs (**O**ne stone) in a 3-month period?

Do you believe yourself to be **F**at when others say you are too thin?

Would you say that **F**ood dominates your life?

Screen for Disordered Eating (Maguen et al. 2018)

Do you often feel the desire to eat when you are emotionally upset or stressed?

Do you often feel that you can't control what or how much you eat?

Do you sometimes make yourself throw up (vomit) to control your weight?

Are you often preoccupied with a desire to be thinner?

Do you believe yourself to be fat when others say you are too thin?

Eating Disorder Screen for Primary Care (Cotton et al. 2003)

Are you satisfied with your eating patterns? (A "no" to this question is classified as an abnormal response.)

Do you ever eat in secret? (A "yes" to this and all other questions is classified as an abnormal response.)

Does your weight affect the way you feel about yourself?

Have any members of your family suffered with an eating disorder?

Do you currently suffer with or have you ever suffered in the past with an eating disorder?

- percentage of time preoccupied with food, weight, and body shape;
- prior treatment and response to treatment for an eating disorder;
- psychosocial impairment secondary to eating or body image concerns or behaviors; and
- family history of eating disorders, other psychiatric illnesses, and other medical conditions (e.g., obesity, inflammatory bowel disease, diabetes mellitus).

Implementation

A careful assessment of the patient's history, symptoms, behaviors, and mental status is the first step in making a diagnosis of an eating disorder. This assessment can take several visits to complete and should also address the recommendations of the *American Psychiatric Association Practice Guidelines for the Psychiatric Evaluation of Adults* (American Psychiatric Association 2016). Information can be obtained through face-to-face interviews, standardized assessment tools, physical examination, laboratory testing, and input from collateral sources, such as family members, other health professionals, and medical records. For a variety of reasons (e.g., ambivalence about changing behavior, stigma, impaired insight), individuals with eating disorders may underreport symptoms (e.g., amount of food consumed, time spent exercising, episodes of binge eating and/or purging). Consequently, family members, partners, or others may observe changes in eating or other behaviors that the patient does not report. In the assessment of children and adolescents, it is essential to involve parents or guardians and, whenever appropriate, school personnel and health professionals who routinely work with the patient. Because many symptoms of eating disorders are cognitive in nature (e.g., fear of weight gain, overvaluation of weight and body shape) and depend on abstract reasoning ability, children may not have the capacity to articulate or endorse such symptoms, and greater reliance on behavioral indicators may be necessary (Lock et al. 2015a). In addition, children and adolescents may exhibit different psychosocial changes than adults as their eating-related symptoms evolve (Hornberger et al. 2021; Lock et al. 2015a). Thus, as a complement to the psychosocial assessment conducted as part of any initial evaluation (American Psychiatric Association 2016), it can be helpful to identify changes in school performance, athletic pursuits, or other differences in psychosocial functioning when assessing children or adolescents with an eating disorder. Clinicians should also keep in mind that the clinical presentation of an eating disorder may be influenced by cultural considerations, although individuals of all age groups, genders, and cultural groups may develop an eating disorder (George and Franko 2010; Hudson et al. 2007; Makino et al. 2004; Perez et al. 2016; Udo and Grilo 2018).

The initial assessment of a patient with a possible eating disorder should include a thorough history of the patient's height and weight, including lifetime maximum and minimum weights. Clinicians should assess the degree of recent weight loss because medical complications (e.g., refeeding syndrome) are predicted by both the rapidity and total magnitude of weight loss (Garber et al. 2019; Whitelaw et al. 2018). Asking the patient about the weight that would be most comfortable for them can help align treatment-planning goals and provide additional useful information about the patient's degree of insight (e.g., if they select a desired weight that is significantly below the normal range). The clinician should also document any changes in adult height because this may reflect bone loss resulting from chronic nutritional deficiency (Misra et al. 2016).

For children and adolescents, obtaining historical height and weight percentiles through growth curves or charts (either documented directly or obtained from the patient's pediatrician or family physician) may help to identify growth retardation associated with AN and is extremely important for characterizing changes in the patient's weight and height trajectory (Marion et al. 2020; Modan-Moses et al. 2003, 2021; Swenne and Thurfjell 2003). It can also be helpful to take a developmental history of feeding and eating, as described below for ARFID.

A thorough assessment of food and eating patterns, and any changes to patterns of eating behavior, is critical for evaluation of a possible eating disorder. Food repertoire changes (as reflected by typical daily diet habits) may include choosing foods with different (often lower) caloric density, changing to a specific type of diet (e.g., vegan/vegetarian, high protein/paleo, gluten free), reducing the variety of foods eaten, avoiding entire food groups (e.g., dairy) or macronutrients (e.g., fat, carbohydrates), or developing food intolerances, phobias, or aversions. Consequently, it is important to determine whether food ingestion is sufficient to sustain healthy growth and development, whether patterns of food restriction or avoidance may contribute to possible nutritional deficiencies, and whether significant changes in food preferences represent onset of health conditions other than eating disorders. It can also be helpful to ask about ways in which patients find eating behaviors to be helpful to them, including their motivations for food restriction or avoidance. Such inquiries can help patients feel understood and can identify gaps in coping strategies that may warrant attention in treatment.

Individuals with eating disorders, particularly individuals with AN (Gianini et al. 2015), may exhibit abnormal mealtime behaviors, such as excessively tearing or cutting up foods, chewing each bite a certain number of times, delaying onset of eating, or avoiding particular combinations of foods. Other eating disorder-related behaviors may include chewing and spitting, rumination, or concern about gastrointestinal (GI) effects of eating (e.g., fullness, bloating, abdominal pain). Individuals with an eating disorder may also avoid social situations because of heightened sensory experiences of others' food, feelings of disgust at watching others eat, or self-consciousness about others commenting on their food choices.

Clinicians should inquire about the presence of binge eating, during which the individual experiences a sense of loss of control over eating and consumes an amount of food that is definitely larger than most people would eat under similar circumstances (American Psychiatric Association 2013). It is helpful to learn what occurs during a patient's typical binge, because their subjective description may provide additional insights into their eating behaviors. Patients should also be asked about purging behavior, which may involve self-induced vomiting or laxative or diuretic use, as well as the frequency of purging behavior, including details on the type and quantity of laxatives or diuretics used and whether there have been recent changes in the pattern and frequency of purging behavior. In addition, clinicians should inquire about compensatory behaviors, such as the use of medication to manipulate weight (e.g., diuretics, caffeine, stimulants, diet pills, nutritional or herbal supplements, muscle building supplements, insulin omission or dose manipulation, thyroid hormones) or excessive exercise. Indicators of compensatory or excessive exercise may include an unwillingness or inability to adapt one's exercise regimen when injured and rigidity and/or preoccupation with one's exercise routine to the extent that it contributes to social avoidance (e.g., being so concerned with waking up to exercise that one does not go out with friends in the evening).

Individuals with a possible eating disorder should be asked about the amount of time they spend preoccupied with thoughts about eating, weight, or body shape. Although not all individuals with an eating disorder will report these features, disturbance in the experience of the body and/or overvaluation of weight and body shape may be reflected in negative subjective evaluations of one's appearance (e.g., feelings of self-disgust toward one's body), body dissatisfaction (including concern with muscle definition or specific body areas), difficulties trusting perceptions of interoceptive and proprioceptive sensations (e.g., not trusting experiences of hunger as real, concerns about GI symptoms), behavioral rituals (e.g., frequent weighing, checking size of body areas), and cognitive preoccupations (e.g., fear of gaining weight, anxiety about eating, disgust with food, concerns about eating in social situations). In men, there can be a greater focus on muscularity rather than weight per se (Lavender et al. 2017). Bullying and cyberbullying are common and may contribute to body dissatisfaction, among other psychological effects (Day et al. 2022; Lie et al. 2019, 2021a, 2021b; Solmi et al. 2021). In addition, it can often be helpful to ask about social media interactions or peer groups influences that affect patients' views of eating, weight, or body shape (Padín et al. 2021; Scott et al. 2019).

In transgender and gender non-binary youth, gender-affirming motivations can lead to dietary restriction or other compensatory behaviors to prevent puberty onset or progression (Avila et al. 2019; Coelho et al. 2019). It is also important to learn whether the patient has had gender-affirming medical interventions, including hormone therapy or surgical interventions, and their association with changes in eating disorder symptoms (Jones et al. 2018; Nowaskie et al. 2021; Uniacke et al. 2021).

Gathering information on prior treatment and treatment response can be helpful in conceptualizing the severity and course of illness and in formulating the initial treatment plan. In addition to treatment settings and levels of care, clinicians should inquire about prior experience with, and response to, both psychotherapeutic and pharmacological interventions. Premorbid personality traits (e.g., perfectionism, conscientiousness, and obsessionality in AN; impulsivity with binge eating or purging behavior) may influence symptom severity, treatment planning, and outcomes for individuals with an eating disorder (Dahlenburg et al. 2019; Dufresne et al. 2020; Hower et al. 2021; Legg and Turner 2021; Lilenfeld et al. 2006; Waxman 2009).

The initial assessment should also include a thorough family history. Patients should be asked about a family history of eating disorders, binge eating, dieting or restrictive eating, obesity, or other weight-related issues as well as about family and cultural attitudes toward eating, exercise, and appearance. Clinicians should also inquire about family history of conditions that may be common in individuals with eating disorders, such as diabetes mellitus, inflammatory bowel disease, and other psychiatric disorders, including depression, anxiety, OCD, and substance use disorders (Hudson et al. 2007). Although asking about a family history of suicide is important in every psychiatric evaluation, it is particularly relevant when evaluating a patient with a possible eating disorder given the elevated rates of suicide in this population (Arcelus et al. 2011). When assessing adolescents, clinicians should also consider the role of family interactions and attitudes (Blissett and Haycraft 2011; Lydecker and Grilo 2016) that may require attention as part of the treatment plan.

A patient's degree of insight and capacity to make a reasoned choice about the need for treatment should be assessed because insight and judgment may be impaired by a constellation of factors, including the effects of restrictive eating on cognition. Eating disorders, especially AN, are also characterized by ambivalence toward treatment because interventions that target disordered eating and weight control behaviors may induce anxiety. Patients who have experienced frequent relapses or an extended history of unsuccessful treatment may feel hopeless about the prospects of improvement. For adolescents, the ability to assess future risk depends on the patient's level of cognitive development and can complicate assessments of insight and capacity.

Avoidant/restrictive food intake disorder

In addition to aspects of the initial evaluation described above for any eating disorder, several aspects of the history are particularly relevant to the identification of ARFID. ARFID was first included in DSM-5 (American Psychiatric Association 2013) and consists of an eating or feeding disturbance associated with avoidance or restriction of food intake, as the name implies. There are diverse and overlapping motivations that contribute to food avoidance/restriction, but examples mentioned in DSM-5-TR (American Psychiatric Association 2022) include "an apparent lack of interest in eating or food; avoidance based on the sensory characteristics of food; [or] concern about aversive consequences of eating" (p. 376). Although these features have been the most investigated, these examples should not preclude a clinician from exploring unique contributions to food avoidance/restriction in an individual patient. In addition, at least one of the following features must be present: "Significant weight loss (or failure to achieve expected weight gain or faltering growth in children), significant nutritional deficiency, dependence on enteral feeding or oral nutritional supplements, [or] marked interference with psychosocial functioning" (p. 376). To fulfill the diagnostic criteria for ARFID, the eating and feeding disturbances cannot be the result of a psychiatric condition (e.g., AN, BN), must exceed the impact on eating/feeding contributed by another medical condition (e.g., GI disease), and cannot be a reflection of culturally related eating practices or food scarcity.

If ARFID is suspected, it is especially helpful to take a developmental history of feeding and eating, which may include early problems with breast or formula feeding; ease of transition to solid foods; the presence of oral-motor difficulties that complicated feeding; and food intolerances or allergies that may contribute to early aversive conditioning of eating. Medical conditions such as gastroesophageal reflux disease, eosinophilic esophagitis, and inflammatory bowel disease can also contribute to eating and feeding difficulties (Day et al. 2022; Fink et al. 2022; Gibson et al. 2021; Murray et al. 2021; Oliveira 2021; J.E. Peters et al. 2022; Robson et al. 2019; Yelencich et al. 2022). A comprehensive developmental history may help parents feel that longstanding difficulties are appreciated by medical professionals. Furthermore, finding a sustained pattern of eating problems can alert the clinician to possible mechanical oral motor problems that have gone undetected.

Assessment of nutritional status and examination of growth trajectories are also important for individuals with possible ARFID (Eddy et al. 2019). In addition to changes in weight or slowing of growth, some youth with ARFID can have consistently low height and weight percentiles as well as associated nutritional deficiencies (Feillet et al. 2019; Schmidt et al. 2021; Yule et al. 2021).

With ARFID, patterns of food avoidance are often chronic rather than reflecting a recent change. In other instances, individuals may have experienced an acute GI or other health condition, but disordered eating patterns persist despite resolution of the original problem. Thus, it can be helpful to ask about patients' motivations for food avoidance and the ways in which food avoidance is helpful to them. For example, food avoidance in individuals with ARFID can be motivated by a fear of aversive consequences of eating such as choking, gagging, allergic reactions, pain, or GI effects (e.g., nausea, vomiting, bloating, constipation, diarrhea). In addition, sensory sensitivity to smells, appearance, texture, taste, and/or temperature of food may reduce the willingness and ability to try new or unfamiliar foods, decrease dietary variety in individuals' food repertoire, and even interfere with willingness to eat familiar foods that are not prepared in a precise fashion. Unlike in AN or BN, individuals with ARFID will often prefer bland starchy foods or foods with higher calorie density, yet their total calorie intake is insufficient for weight gain. For some individuals with ARFID, the introduction of a new taste or an unexpected experience with a familiar taste can result in gagging and subsequent avoidance. As with other eating disorders, individuals with ARFID may be uncomfortable with or unable to eat around other people. Meals may terminate prematurely due to low appetitive drive or to avoid eating unfamiliar food, minimize uncomfortable physical sensations (e.g., gut fullness), or escape uncomfortable social eating situations. They may also feel disgust at watching others eat or experience heightened sensory experiences or disgust toward the smell of others' food. Importantly, patients with ARFID vary in their clinical presentations (Katzman et al. 2021; Norris et al. 2018), and understanding the patient's experiences with food can help in establishing rapport as well as serve as a starting point for treatment.

STATEMENT 3: Quantitative Measures

APA *recommends* **(1C)** that the initial psychiatric evaluation of a patient with a possible eating disorder include weighing the patient and quantifying eating and weight control behaviors (e.g., frequency, intensity, or time spent on dietary restriction, binge eating, purging, exercise, and other compensatory behaviors).

Implementation

In the assessment of a patient with a possible eating disorder, obtaining the patient's weight and quantifying recent or current eating and weight control behaviors can help detect and determine the severity of eating disorder behaviors and associated symptoms. Height should also be obtained, as described in Statement 6.

APA's *Practice Guidelines for the Psychiatric Evaluation of Adults*, 3rd Edition (American Psychiatric Association 2016) provides a general description of the use of quantitative measures, which can include use of formal rating scales or quantifying the number or characteristics of relevant behaviors. The intent of using a quantitative measure is not to establish a diagnosis but rather to complement other aspects of the screening and assessment process. Depending on the measure, it can aid in treatment planning by providing a structured, replicable way to document the patient's baseline symptoms. It can also help to determine which symptoms should be the target of intervention based on factors such as frequency of occurrence, magnitude, associated distress to the patient, and potential for associated harm to the patient or others. On the other hand, it is important to be mindful of the fact that some individuals will underreport symptoms, particularly if they do not feel comfortable with the therapeutic relationship, are not motivated for treatment, lack awareness of having a disorder, wish to avoid disappointing the clinician, feel shame about their behavior, or have experienced prior bullying or criticism for their behavior, weight, or appearance.

As treatment proceeds, use of quantitative measures will often allow more precise tracking of whether pharmacological, psychotherapeutic, and other nonpharmacological treatments are having their intended effects or whether a shift in the treatment plan is needed. Standardized assessments can be useful for demonstrating improvement to patients who may feel unmotivated or disappointed with their response to treatment. They can also provide helpful information about the actual effects of prior treatments. Again, however, underreporting may occur, or rates of symptom reporting may increase as motivation to change or insight improve with treatment. In addition, patients' ratings can be compared with family members' impressions of treatment effects to clarify the longitudinal course of the patient's illness.

One approach to quantitative assessment is to focus on measures of eating disorder severity as described in DSM-5 criteria (i.e., weight loss for AN, episodes of inappropriate compensatory behaviors per week for BN, binge-eating episodes per week for BED). In addition to behavior frequency, measures of behavioral intensity or time spent on dietary restriction, binge eating, purging, exercise, and other compensatory behaviors can also be obtained. Weight is a key measure in individuals with an eating disorder and should be obtained with patients dressed in light clothing and with shoes removed. Whether the measured weight should be shared with the patient or not is unclear and may depend on the treatment approach being used as well as patient-specific considerations.

Although use of an eating disorder rating scale is not necessary to quantify eating and weight control behaviors, a number of patient- and clinician-rated scales and screening tools for eating disorders have been developed and validated (Schaefer et al. 2021). If a scale is used, the choice of a scale should consider the age of the patient, clinical setting, time available for administration, and therapeutic objective (i.e., screening vs. diagnosis vs. ongoing monitoring). As discussed in Statement 1, the SCOFF questionnaire is a five-item tool for eating disorders that has high sensitivity and specificity for identifying AN and BN when screening for an eating disorder (Kutz et al. 2020; Morgan et al. 1999). The Eating Disorder Assessment for DSM-5 (EDA-5) is a freely available clinician-rated, semistructured interview that shows good reliability for diagnosis of AN, BN, and BED in adolescents and adults (www.eda5.org; Sysko et al. 2015). It also has a youth version available for ages 8–14 as well as versions in Spanish and other languages. The Eating Disorders Examination Questionnaire (EDE-Q) is a relatively brief, freely available, and well-validated self-report measure that is adapted from the semistructured Eating Disorders Examination (EDE) interview (Fairburn 2008). It has been validated in Spanish (Grilo et al. 2012a; Peláez-Fernández et al. 2012) and multiple other languages (Lichtenstein et al. 2021). It may have lower validity in men (Smith et al. 2017), but it appears to be a useful self-report measure in transgender and gender-diverse individuals, although further validation is warranted (Avila et al. 2019; Duffy et al. 2021; Nagata et al. 2020a, 2020c; Nowaskie et al. 2021). The EDE-Q is reliable in adults as well as in adolescents (Mond et al. 2004; Schaefer et al. 2018), and a children's version of the EDE-Q has been validated for use in 7- to 18-year-olds (Kliem et al. 2017). Another scale developed for children and adolescents ages 8–14 years is the Kids' Eating Disorders Survey (Brewerton 2001; Childress et al. 1993). For assessing longitudinal changes in eating-related cognitions and behaviors, the Eating Disorders 15 (ED-15) has been developed (Tatham et al. 2015) and has a corresponding version for youth (Accurso and Waller 2021a) and for reporting by parents or caregivers (Accurso and Waller 2021b). The Clinical Impairment Assessment (CIA; www.psytoolkit.org/survey-library/eating-cia.html) is a self-report measure available in English and Spanish to measure psychosocial impairment associated with an eating disorder (Bohn et al. 2008; Jenkins 2013; Maraldo et al. 2021; Martín et al. 2015; Raykos et al. 2019), although different thresholds for total scores may be needed in men and women (Richson et al. 2021).

For assessment of other disorders related to eating, the Eating Disorders in Youth Questionnaire has been validated for use in 8- to 13-year-olds (Goldberg et al. 2020) and the Nine Item Avoidant/Restrictive Food Intake Disorder Screen (Zickgraf and Ellis 2018) has been validated for use in adults. The Pica, ARFID, and Rumination Disorder Interview (PARDI; Bryant-Waugh et al. 2019) is a multi-informant, semistructured instrument that is used in research; however, clinicians may benefit from reviewing the items on the PARDI to learn about clinical features of these disorders.

STATEMENT 4: Identification of Co-Occurring Conditions

APA *recommends* (1C) that the initial psychiatric evaluation of a patient with a possible eating disorder identify co-occurring health conditions, including co-occurring psychiatric disorders.

Implementation

Co-occurring health conditions are important to identify as part of the evaluation of a patient with a possible eating disorder. Some co-occurring health conditions may be a sequela of an eating disorder (e.g., gastroesophageal reflux disease, irritable bowel syndrome, gastroparesis, other GI motility disorders), whereas others (e.g., diabetes mellitus, celiac disease, inflammatory bowel disease) can place restrictions on eating behaviors and dietary variety and can exacerbate or increase the likelihood of developing an eating disorder (Nikniaz et al. 2021; J.E. Peters et al. 2022; Young et al. 2013). Even when a health condition is independent of an eating disorder, it can influence the choice of treatment or a need for medical stabilization.

Identification of preexisting or co-occurring psychiatric conditions and obtaining information on their onset and course is also important for treatment planning. When another psychiatric condition is present, outcomes are worse (Franko et al. 2018; Keshishian et al. 2019; Lydecker and Grilo 2021; Riquin et al. 2021) and mortality is greater (Himmerich et al. 2019a, 2019b; Kask et al. 2016, 2017). Thus, it is essential to provide care for both the eating disorder and other psychiatric conditions. The relationship between eating disorders and psychiatric symptoms is complex; careful clinical assessment is needed to discern whether symptoms of depression, anxiety, or obsessionality reflect an independent co-occurring disorder or have developed as a result of the eating disorder. For example, starvation has been shown to lead to depressive symptoms, including low mood, impaired concentration, low energy, and sleep disturbance, as well as increased anxiety and obsessionality (Keys et al. 1950). On the other hand, eating disorders frequently co-occur with other psychiatric disorders, particularly depression, anxiety, OCD, PTSD, autism spectrum disorder, substance use disorders, and personality disorders (Hudson et al. 2007; Steinhausen et al. 2021). Individuals with an eating disorder also have a greater likelihood of ADHD than individuals without an eating disorder (Brewerton and Duncan 2016; Nazar et al. 2016). Physical restlessness is commonly observed in low-weight patients with AN and can manifest as persistent fidgeting or refusal to sit for extended periods of time, independent of the presence of ADHD.

A history of trauma may also increase risk for development of disordered eating behaviors (Emery et al. 2021; Russon et al. 2019) or an eating disorder. Reports of prior sexual trauma are elevated in patients with eating disorders (Lie et al. 2021a; Madowitz et al. 2015; Solmi et al. 2021), but rates of physical or emotional abuse or neglect are also increased (Afifi et al. 2017; Coffino et al. 2020; Hazzard et al. 2019; Kimber et al. 2017; Lie et al. 2021a; Molendijk et al. 2017; Pignatelli et al. 2017). In addition, many individuals who have an eating disorder have experienced bullying or criticism of their weight or appearance (Day et al. 2022; Lie et al. 2019, 2021b; Solmi et al. 2021). Consequently, all patients with a possible eating disorder should be asked about a history of trauma; physical, emotional, or sexual abuse; bullying (including cyberbullying); or neglect (including food insecurity) and assessed for symptoms related to PTSD (Ferrell et al. 2020).

Suicide is the second leading cause of death among individuals with AN, and rates of suicidal behavior are elevated in individuals with BN and BED (Smith et al. 2018). The initial examination should include a thorough assessment of suicide risk, including current suicidal ideas, plans, or intentions, prior suicidal plans or attempts, and the presence of non-suicidal self-injury (see Guideline III, "Assessment of Suicide Risk," in the APA's *Practice Guidelines for the Psychiatric Evaluation of Adults*; American Psychiatric Association 2016). Such assessments can be conducted through clinical interview, mental status examination, or use of quantitative measures.

For any patient who is undergoing an initial psychiatric evaluation, it is important to assess the patient's use of caffeine, tobacco, alcohol, cannabinoids, and other substances, as well as any misuse of prescribed or over-the-counter (OTC) medications or supplements (see Guideline II, "Substance Use Assessment," in the *Practice Guidelines for the Psychiatric Evaluation of Adults*; American Psychiatric Association 2016). Substance use disorders are frequently comorbid with eating disorders (Bahji et al. 2019; Harrop and Marlatt 2010; Javaras et al. 2008; Krug et al. 2008); thus, a comprehensive substance use history is essential in a patient with a potential eating disorder. Cigarette smoking (including electronic cigarettes or vaping) can be used to suppress appetite (Mason et al. 2021; Naveed et al. 2021), and smoking can affect the rate of weight restoration during treatment (Van Wymelbeke et al. 2004). A specific inquiry should also be made about the use or misuse of prescribed or non-prescribed medications that suppress appetite (e.g., OTC weight loss products, stimulants) or enhance muscularity (e.g., supplements, androgens).

Among individuals with ARFID, comorbidity with GI disease (e.g., achalasia, eosinophilic esophagitis, celiac disease, inflammatory bowel disease) is common (Day et al. 2022; Fink et al. 2022; Gibson et al. 2021; Murray et al. 2021; J.E. Peters et al. 2022; Robson et al. 2019; Yelencich et al. 2022) and evaluation for GI abnormalities may be warranted, particularly in individuals whose symptoms are not lifelong. Autism spectrum disorder and ADHD also appear to be more frequent in individuals with ARFID (Farag et al. 2022; Keery et al. 2019; Yule et al. 2021), emphasizing the importance of taking a history for developmental, learning, and sensory issues. Anxiety symptoms and diagnoses (Fisher et al. 2014; Kambanis et al. 2020; Katzman et al. 2021; Keery et al. 2019; Norris et al. 2014, 2021) and depressive symptoms (Katzman et al. 2021) are also reported frequently by individuals with ARFID. More detailed recommendations about screening for co-occurring conditions can be found in the *Practice Guidelines for the Psychiatric Evaluation of Adults* (American Psychiatric Association 2016).

STATEMENT 5: Initial Review of Systems

APA *recommends* **(1C)** that the initial psychiatric evaluation of a patient with a possible eating disorder include a comprehensive review of systems.

Implementation

The effects of malnutrition, binge eating, and purging can affect every organ system in the body (Academy for Eating Disorders Medical Care Standards Committee 2021; Cass et al. 2020; Sachs and Mehler 2016). In addition to the recommendations for a review of systems as found in the *Practice Guidelines for the Psychiatric Evaluation of Adults* (American Psychiatric Association 2016), a focus on issues that are common in patients with eating disorders can help to identify preexisting or co-occurring conditions (as discussed in Statement 4) as well as elicit symptoms of concern to the patient (see Table 3). Although some of these symptoms or conditions may improve or resolve with treatment of the eating disorder, others will require additional evaluation and treatment in addition to treatment of the eating disorder.

Patients with eating disorders commonly report symptoms such as abdominal discomfort or pain with eating, constipation, early satiety or fullness, bloating, nausea, and gastroesophageal reflux (Riedlinger et al. 2020). These symptoms do not necessarily reflect evidence of a structural GI disorder but may be a consequence of starvation and disordered eating patterns that result in functional GI disorders and problems with GI motility (e.g., delayed gastric emptying [Hetterich et al. 2019]). Patients who induce vomiting should be asked about hematemesis.

Cardiovascular issues are also common as described further in Statement 8. Changes in cardiac rhythm include bradycardia, whereas other arrhythmias can present with palpitations (Giovinazzo et al. 2019; Sachs et al. 2016). Low blood pressure, often in association with orthostatic hypotension, can result in dizziness on standing or syncope. Rates of mitral valve prolapse, pericardial effusion, and myocardial atrophy also appear to be increased in individuals with AN (Giovinazzo et al. 2019; Olivares et al. 2005; Sachs et al. 2016; Smythe et al. 2021).

It is similarly important to inquire about past or current neurological signs or symptoms, such as seizures and headache (including migraine headaches). Osteoporosis and fractures (including stress fractures) occur at an increased frequency in individuals with an eating disorder (Frölich et al. 2020; Robinson et al. 2016, 2019; Solmi et al. 2016) and should also be identified as part of the review of systems.

Assessment should include taking a menstrual history, when relevant, including age of menarche and date of last menstrual period. It is also important to ask about use of oral contraceptives or other hormonal therapies that may affect menses. Menstrual cycle abnormalities, including irregular periods and amenorrhea, occur in AN (Misra and Klibanski 2014), atypical AN (Garber et al. 2019; Lebow et al. 2015; Rastogi et al. 2020), BN (Gendall et al. 2000), and BED (Olguin et al. 2017). In addition, polycystic ovary syndrome also appears to be associated with an increased likelihood of having disordered eating (Pirotta et al. 2019) or an eating disorder, particularly BN or BED (Thannickal et al. 2020). Dietary restriction with significant weight reduction or a low BMI can also be associated with increased rates of pregnancy complications and neonatal difficulties. Patients should be asked about sexual (e.g., decrease in libido, erectile dysfunction) and reproductive (e.g., infertil-

TABLE 3. Signs and symptoms of eating disorders

Organ system	Symptom/*Sign*[1]	
	Related to nutritional restriction	**Related to purging**
General	*Low weight, cachexia*	
General	Fatigue	
General	*Weakness*	*Weakness*
General	*Dehydration*	
General	Cold intolerance, *low body temperature*	
General	Hot flashes, sweating	
Nervous system	Anxiety, depression, or irritability	Anxiety, depression, or irritability
Nervous system	Apathy	Apathy
Nervous system	Poor concentration	Poor concentration
Nervous system	Headache	Headache
Nervous system	*Seizures* (in severe cases)	*Seizures* (in severe cases)
Nervous system		Paresthesia (due to electrolyte abnormalities)
Nervous system	*Peripheral polyneuropathy* (in severe cases)	
Oropharyngeal	Dysphagia	
Oropharyngeal		*Dental enamel erosion and decay*
Oropharyngeal		*Enlarged salivary glands*
Oropharyngeal		Pharyngeal pain
Oropharyngeal		*Palatal scratches, erythema, or petechiae*
Gastrointestinal	Abdominal discomfort	Abdominal discomfort
Gastrointestinal	Constipation	Constipation
Gastrointestinal		Diarrhea (due to laxative use)
Gastrointestinal	Nausea	
Gastrointestinal	Early satiety	
Gastrointestinal	*Abdominal distention*, bloating	*Abdominal distention*, bloating
Gastrointestinal		Heartburn, *gastroesophageal erosions or inflammation*
Gastrointestinal		*Vomiting, possibly blood-streaked*
Gastrointestinal		*Rectal prolapse*
Cardiovascular	Dizziness, faintness, *orthostatic hypotension*	Dizziness, faintness, *orthostatic hypotension*
Cardiovascular	Palpitations, *arrhythmias*	Palpitations, *arrhythmias*
Cardiovascular	*Bradycardia*	
Cardiovascular	*Weak irregular pulse*	
Cardiovascular	*Cold extremities, acrocyanosis*	
Cardiovascular	Chest pain	
Cardiovascular	*Dyspnea*	
Reproductive/Endocrine	*Slowing of growth (in children or adolescents)*	*Slowing of growth (in children or adolescents)*
Reproductive/Endocrine	*Arrested development of secondary sex characteristics*	*Arrested development of secondary sex characteristics*
Reproductive/Endocrine	Low libido	Low libido
Reproductive/Endocrine	*Fertility problems*	
Reproductive/Endocrine	*Oligomenorrhea*	*Oligomenorrhea*
Reproductive/Endocrine	*Primary or secondary amenorrhea*	
Musculoskeletal	*Proximal muscle weakness, wasting, or atrophy*	
Musculoskeletal		Muscle cramping

TABLE 3. Signs and symptoms of eating disorders *(continued)*

| | Symptom/*Sign*[1] | |
Organ system	Related to nutritional restriction	Related to purging
Musculoskeletal	Bone pain[2]	Bone pain[2]
Musculoskeletal	*Stress fractures*[2]	*Stress fractures*[2]
Musculoskeletal	*Slowed growth (relative to expected)*[2]	*Slowed growth (relative to expected)*[2]
Dermatological	*Dry, yellow skin*	
Dermatological	*Change in hair including hair loss and dry and brittle hair*	
Dermatological	*Lanugo*	
Dermatological		*Scarring on dorsum of hand (Russell's sign)*
Dermatological	*Poor skin turgor*	*Poor skin turgor*
Dermatological	*Pitting edema (with refeeding)*	*Pitting edema*

Note. [1]Symptoms are in roman font; signs are in italic font.
[2]Risk of skeletal effects is in individuals with previous low weight and menstrual irregularity or amenorrhea.

ity, obstetrical complications) issues that may arise in the setting of altered hypothalamic-pituitary-gonadal axis functioning.

STATEMENT 6: Initial Physical Examination

APA *recommends* (1C) that the initial physical examination of a patient with a possible eating disorder include assessment of vital signs, including temperature, resting heart rate, blood pressure, orthostatic pulse, and orthostatic blood pressure; height, weight, and BMI (or percent median BMI, BMI percentile, or BMI Z-score for children and adolescents); and physical appearance, including signs of malnutrition or purging behaviors.

Implementation

A complete physical examination is strongly recommended in addition to assessment of vital signs and physical appearance. As described in the *Practice Guidelines for the Psychiatric Evaluation of Adults* (American Psychiatric Association 2016), it may be performed by a psychiatrist, another physician, or a medically trained clinician but is best performed by a clinician familiar with common findings in patients with eating disorders. Diagnosis should rely on a comprehensive assessment of psychiatric and medical status and history because a physical examination with normal results may not exclude an eating disorder. Furthermore, physical findings such as low blood pressure or low resting heart rate, which can be seen in healthy individuals, may not be a marker of health in an individual with other evidence of an eating disorder. Following the initial evaluation, the frequency of physical assessment will depend on the individual's clinical status.

Table 2 describes physical signs that may occur in individuals with an eating disorder. The physical examination should give particular attention to vital signs because abnormalities may indicate medical instability, which would warrant a higher level of care (see Statement 9). Abnormalities of potential concern include a heart rate <50 beats per minute (bpm), a systolic blood pressure <90 mmHg, or a temperature <36°C (96.8°F). A sustained decrease of systolic blood pressure of at least 20 mmHg or pulse increases of >30 bpm in adults or >40 bpm in adolescents ages 12–19 years within 3 minutes from lying to standing may also indicate medical instability (Freeman et al. 2011; Raj et al. 2020; Singer et al. 2012). All patients should be evaluated for evidence of self-injurious behaviors because individuals with eating disorders experience elevated rates of self-injury compared to the general population (Cucchi et al. 2016; Forrest et al. 2021; Kostro et al. 2014). Physical examination of children and adolescents with a possible eating disorder should also include assessment of growth and pubertal development (e.g., as indicated by the Tanner stage of sexual maturity).

Patient height, weight, and BMI should be evaluated initially, with weight obtained, ideally, at all visits (see www.cdc.gov/healthyweight/assessing/bmi/adult_bmi/english_bmi_calculator/ bmi_calculator.html). The frequency at which the patient's height needs to be measured will vary, with adults requiring height determinations less frequently than adolescents. Some patients may prefer to be weighed in a blinded fashion (i.e., turn around to remain unaware of their weight; Froreich et al. 2020; Wagner et al. 2013). The decision to weigh patients in this manner as compared to an open fashion is controversial and often depends on the philosophy of the eating disorders treatment program. Other factors that may influence the choice of blinded as compared to open weighing can include the type of setting (inpatient vs. outpatient), the type of psychotherapy (e.g., family-based therapy [FBT], cognitive-behavioral therapy [CBT]), the frequency of weight checks, and patient characteristics or preferences (Forbush et al. 2015). Even when weighing does occur in a blinded fashion, patients may become aware of their weight through electronic health record notes.

When interpreting a patient's BMI and related measures, it is important to be aware of the limitations of this parameter. In particular, it does not distinguish between fat and muscle mass, reflect differences in fat distribution, or incorporate variations in BMI due to age, sex, race, or ethnicity (Kesztyüs et al. 2021; Lee et al. 2017; Liu et al. 2021; Tinsley et al. 2020). Nevertheless, it is readily measurable and in frequent clinical and research use. In children and adolescents, percent median BMI (current BMI/50th percentile BMI for age and sex×100; www.cdc.gov/healthyweight/bmi/ calculator.html), BMI percentile, or BMI Z-score should be determined (Golden et al. 2015a). Longitudinal growth charts should be documented directly or obtained from the patient's pediatrician or family physician to assess for deviations from individual growth trajectories and to guide determination of a target weight. Such an approach can also help to identify growth retardation associated with AN (Marion et al. 2020; Modan-Moses et al. 2003, 2021; Swenne and Thurfjell 2003), weight suppression in association with atypical AN, or consistently low height and weight percentiles as can be seen in some youth with ARFID (Yule et al. 2021).

Patients should be evaluated for physical manifestations of malnutrition, which may include proximal muscle and temporal wasting, ankle and pedal edema, and dermatological changes such as lanugo (fine downy hair), hair loss, and dry skin. In addition, some individuals with severe dietary restriction may become immunocompromised (Brown et al. 2008). Signs of malnutrition improve with normalization of eating behavior and weight; targeted treatment (e.g., use of diuretics for malnutrition-related peripheral edema) is rarely needed for these signs.

Vitamin deficiencies (e.g., vitamin A, thiamine, vitamin B_{12}, vitamin C, vitamin D, zinc) can also develop due to dietary restrictions in individuals with AN, atypical AN, or ARFID (Achamrah et al. 2017; Hanachi et al. 2019; Yule et al. 2021). Risk of vitamin deficiencies can be compounded by co-occurring conditions (e.g., thiamine deficiency with co-occurring alcohol use disorder). Physical findings may include angular stomatitis, glossitis, bleeding gums, and dermatological, ocular, or neurological findings (Suter and Russell 2018).

Clinicians should also assess for any signs of purging, such as parotid gland enlargement, dental enamel erosion, and calluses on the knuckles or dorsum of the hand (Russell's sign) from scraping against the teeth during attempts to induce vomiting. If purging behavior is present, referral for a dental evaluation is indicated. Although seemingly paradoxical, patients should be instructed not to brush teeth after vomiting (Meurman and ten Cate 1996; Otsu et al. 2014). Oral rinsing with water after vomiting and avoiding ingestion of carbonated beverages or citrus fruits may also help to reduce effects on dentition (Otsu et al. 2014).

STATEMENT 7: Initial Laboratory Assessment

APA *recommends* **(1C)** that the laboratory assessment of a patient with a possible eating disorder include a complete blood count and a comprehensive metabolic panel, including electrolytes, liver enzymes, and renal function tests.

Implementation

Laboratory assessments can be helpful in the initial assessment of a patient with a possible eating disorder in detecting abnormalities that may require intervention (see Table 4), including a higher level of care. Abnormalities are more frequent in individuals with severe or chronic illness, frequent purging behaviors, or rapid recent weight loss, independent of the individual's current weight. On the other hand, abnormal laboratory values do not occur in all individuals with an eating disorder, and normal laboratory values do not rule out a potential eating disorder.

Patients with eating disorders, particularly those who are at low weight, may present with anemia, leukopenia, and/or thrombocytopenia (Cleary et al. 2010; Hütter et al. 2009; Peebles and Sieke 2019). In individuals who purge or restrict fluids, hemoconcentration resulting from dehydration may initially mask anemia. These hematological abnormalities are typically reversible with restoration to a normal weight. Individuals with AN may show evidence of hepatic dysfunction (Rosen et al. 2016), reflected by elevations in liver enzymes (alanine aminotransferase [ALT] and aspartate aminotransferase [AST]). A rise in aminotransferases may also occur in conjunction with renourishment due to hepatic steatosis (Rosen et al. 2016). Patients with AN may also develop hypoglycemia in the setting of reduced glycogen stores and impaired gluconeogenesis (Gaudiani et al. 2012). In addition, postprandial hypoglycemia can occur in individuals with a low BMI (Hart et al. 2011; Kinzig et al. 2007). Electrolyte disturbances are common and can result from restrictive eating, purging, or laxative or diuretic use. Individuals who vomit regularly can develop hypokalemia and hypochloremic metabolic alkalosis, whereas patients who misuse laxatives may develop a hyperchloremic metabolic acidosis (Peebles and Sieke 2019). Although less common, patients with eating disorders who drink excessive amounts of water may present with hyponatremia, which poses a risk for seizures (Miller et al. 2005). The risk of hyponatremia may also be increased by concurrent use of medications that can cause it (e.g., SSRIs). Measurement of urinary specific gravity can help to identify individuals who are consuming excess water or, conversely, are at risk of dehydration. When volume depletion is severe, such as in individuals with AN who also purge, increases in blood urea nitrogen (BUN) and creatinine can be seen and, rarely, renal failure may occur.

The need for additional laboratory analyses should be determined on an individual basis depending on the patient's condition or the laboratory tests' relevance to making treatment decisions. Serum magnesium and phosphorus levels are commonly measured and may need to be ordered separately from a comprehensive metabolic panel. They should be considered depending on the patient's clinical picture (e.g., risk of refeeding complications, low BMI, rapid recent weight loss, significant medical comorbidities, severe malnourishment). The risk of abnormal magnesium and phosphorus levels is not limited to low-weight individuals with eating disorders; hypomagnesemia can develop in patients with purging behavior (Raj et al. 2012), whereas hypophosphatemia can emerge in individuals with erratic eating patterns (e.g., periods of severe restriction or fasting behavior). Serum amylase levels, specifically levels of salivary amylase, may be elevated in patients who self-induce vomiting. With starvation and with renourishment, elevations in serum lipase can be seen but generally do not require intervention.

Individuals with AN have reduced bone mineral density (BMD) and increased fracture risk (Faje et al. 2014; Lucas et al. 1999; Misra et al. 2008a, 2008b; Nagata et al. 2017; Vestergaard et al. 2003). Prolonged amenorrhea is associated with reduced BMD. Thus, in patients with menstrual irregularities and primary or secondary amenorrhea, gonadotropin (e.g., follicle stimulating hormone, luteinizing hormone), estradiol, and prolactin levels can be measured, as well as a urine pregnancy

TABLE 4. Laboratory abnormalities related to nutritional restriction or purging behaviors

	Organ system	Test	Related to nutritional restriction	Related to purging
Recommended	Cardiovascular	ECG	Bradycardia or arrhythmias, QTc prolongation	Increased P-wave amplitude and duration, increased PR interval, widened QRS complex, QTc prolongation, ST depression, T-wave inversion or flattening, U waves, supraventricular or ventricular tachyarrhythmias
Recommended	Metabolic	Serum electrolytes	Hypokalemia, hyponatremia, hypomagnesemia, hypophosphatemia (especially on refeeding)	Hypokalemia, hyponatremia, hypochloremia, hypomagnesemia, hypophosphatemia, metabolic acidosis
		Lipid panel	Hypercholesterolemia	
		Serum glucose	Low blood sugar	
Recommended	Gastrointestinal	Liver function and associated tests	Elevated liver function tests	
Recommended	Genitourinary	Renal function tests	Increased BUN, decreased GFR, decreased Cr because of low lean body mass (normal Cr may indicate azotemia), renal failure (rare)	Increased BUN and Cr, renal failure (rare)
Based on history or exam	Genitourinary	Urinalysis	Urinary specific gravity abnormalities	Urinary specific gravity abnormalities, high pH
Based on history or exam	Reproductive	Serum gonadotropins and sex hormones	Decreased serum estrogen or serum testosterone; prepubertal patterns of luteinizing hormone, follicle stimulating hormone secretion	May be hypoestrogenemic, if menstrual irregularities are present
Based on history or exam	Skeletal	Bone densitometry (DXA scan)	Reduced BMD, osteopenia, or osteoporosis in individuals with previous low weight and menstrual irregularity or amenorrhea	Reduced BMD, osteopenia, or osteoporosis in individuals with previous low weight and menstrual irregularity or amenorrhea
Incidental	Oropharyngeal	Dental radiography		Erosion of dental enamel

Note. BMD=bone mineral density; BUN=blood urea nitrogen; Cr=creatinine; DXA=Dual-energy X-ray absorptiometry; ECG= electrocardiogram; GFR=glomerular filtration rate; QTc=corrected QT interval.

test (American College of Obstetricians and Gynecologists 2018). Testosterone levels also appear to influence bone density in individuals of all genders (Khosla and Monroe 2018). Some groups have recommended based on consensus that, after 6 months of amenorrhea, bone densitometry (dual-energy X-ray absorptiometry [DXA] scan) may be warranted (Golden et al. 2014, 2015b; Gordon et al. 2017). Other clinicians obtain a DXA scan as a baseline measure even in patients with regular menses. In non-menstruating individuals with AN, there are no data to inform decisions about when to order a DXA scan. In all patients, evidence of low BMD can be useful in providing education about the health impact of AN and motivating them to gain weight.

Measurement of thyroid stimulating hormone can serve as a screening test for possible misuse of thyroid hormone (e.g., OTC thyroid supplements or levothyroxine) and can help rule out other medical conditions such as hyperthyroidism, which can lead to weight loss. On the other hand, individuals who have had significant weight loss and malnutrition can exhibit a nonthyroidal illness syndrome in which levels of total T3 are low and levels of thyroid stimulating hormone may be normal or reduced (Schorr and Miller 2017).

Other potentially useful laboratory assessments include a urine toxicology screen to assist in identifying stimulant misuse, measurement of the erythrocyte sedimentation rate to help distinguish an eating disorder from other inflammatory conditions in patients who report abdominal discomfort after eating, and serum tests to assess for nutritional status or vitamin deficiency (e.g., vitamin D, calcium, iron, thiamine).

STATEMENT 8: Initial Electrocardiogram

APA *recommends* (1C) that an electrocardiogram be done in patients with a restrictive eating disorder, patients with severe purging behavior, and patients who are taking medications that are known to prolong QTc intervals.

Implementation

The appropriateness of an electrocardiogram (ECG) depends on the diagnosis, illness severity, and vital signs and need not be obtained in every patient or in those with mild symptoms. However, an ECG should be obtained in certain circumstances, including for individuals taking medications known to prolong QTc intervals and for those with a restrictive eating disorder, including AN, atypical AN, and ARFID. In addition, patients often underreport purging severity, and obtaining an ECG can identify concerning cardiac changes that may point to an underlying eating disorder.

Individuals with AN are at elevated risk for a number of structural and functional cardiac abnormalities, including bradycardia, myocardial atrophy, pericardial and valvular pathology, conduction abnormalities, and sudden cardiac death (Olivares et al. 2005; Sachs et al. 2016). Less is known about cardiac effects in individuals with atypical AN and ARFID, but bradycardia does occur (Sawyer et al. 2016; Strandjord et al. 2015; Whitelaw et al. 2014, 2018) and may be associated with greater amounts of recent and total weight loss (Whitelaw et al. 2018). In individuals with BN or the binge/purge subtype of AN, self-induced vomiting and/or laxative abuse contribute to an increased risk for prolonged QTc intervals and cardiac arrhythmias due to electrolyte abnormalities (e.g., hypokalemia, metabolic alkalosis; Gibson et al. 2019; Peebles et al. 2010). The risk of QTc prolongation can be increased by concurrent use of medications known to prolong the QT interval. Drug-drug interactions that increase serum levels of these medications can further increase risk. Such medications include, but are not limited to, antidepressants, antipsychotics, antiarrhythmics, some classes of antibiotics (e.g., macrolides, fluoroquinolones), antiviral medications (e.g., for HIV), antiemetics (e.g., ondansetron), antihistamines (e.g., hydroxyzine, diphenhydramine), and some cancer therapeutic agents (Funk et al. 2018; Woosley et al. 2022).

STATEMENT 9: Treatment Plan, Including Level of Care

APA *recommends* (1C) that patients with an eating disorder have a documented, comprehensive, culturally appropriate, and person-centered treatment plan that incorporates medical, psychiatric, psychological, and nutritional expertise, commonly via a coordinated multidisciplinary team.

Implementation

In treating individuals with an eating disorder, a person-centered treatment plan should be developed, documented in the medical record (e.g., as part of a progress note), and updated at appropriate intervals. The aim of person-centered care, which is sometimes referred to as patient-centered care, is to provide care that is respectful of and responsive to individual preferences, needs, and values and ensures that an individual's values guide clinical decisions (Institute of Medicine Committee on Quality of Health Care in America 2001). Person-centered care is achieved through a dynamic and collaborative relationship among individuals, families, other persons of support, and treating clinicians that helps achieve the individual's realistic health and life goals and informs decision-making to the extent that the individual desires (American Geriatrics Society Expert Panel on Person-Centered Care 2016). With person-centered care, patients, families, and other persons of support are provided with information that allows them to make informed decisions (Institute of Medicine 2006). Evidence-based interventions should be adapted to meet individual needs and preferences when possible (van Dulmen et al. 2015). Self-management approaches and shared decision-making are encouraged (Institute of Medicine 2006), with the recognition that shared decision-making may not be possible if an individual lacks awareness of their illness or the need for treatment.

A person-centered treatment plan can be recorded as part of an evaluation note or progress note and does not need to adhere to a defined development process (e.g., face-to-face multidisciplinary team meeting) or format (e.g., time-specified goals and objectives). However, it should give an overview of the identified clinical and psychosocial issues, along with a specific plan for addressing factors such as food avoidance, restrictive eating, binge eating, purging, or other compensatory behaviors (if present) and related social avoidance and/or isolation. The plan should also discuss whether there is a need for further history and mental status examination; physical examination (by either the evaluating clinician or another health professional); laboratory testing; ongoing monitoring; and pharmacological, psychotherapeutic, and other nonpharmacological interventions, as indicated. In addition, the clinical evaluation should include discussion of the patient's gender and their individual strengths, vulnerabilities, personality traits, developmental stage, and motivation for treatment, each of which can inform treatment planning and help anticipate possible issues that may arise during treatment. Collateral informants such as family members, friends, or other treating health professionals may express specific concerns about the individual's eating disorder symptoms. If present, such concerns should be documented and addressed as part of the treatment plan. Treatment plans can also include elements such as collaborating with other treating clinicians, providing integrated care, educating patients about treatment options, discussing the potential impact of social media use on symptoms and eating-related behaviors, engaging family members, exploring family attitudes toward eating, and addressing these attitudes, if indicated.

An understanding of the individual's cultural identity is essential to appreciating the ways in which the patient defines key concerns and values, interacts with family members, receives support from their social network, copes with stressors, and engages in help-seeking behaviors. Cultural and religious beliefs can also be relevant to the patient's dietary choices. The DSM-5-TR Cultural Formulation Interview (American Psychiatric Association 2022) provides a framework for eliciting such information.

Depending on the urgency of the initial clinical presentation, the availability of laboratory results, or receipt of history from collateral informants, the initial treatment plan may need to be augmented over several visits and as more details of the history and treatment response are obtained. The patient's goals and readiness to change eating patterns and behaviors will likely evolve over time. Changes to the treatment plan will also be needed if a patient has not tolerated or responded to a specific treatment or chooses to switch treatment approaches. Symptoms of the eating disorder or of co-occurring conditions may also shift with time and can require a reassessment of the diagnosis or treatment plan.

In determining a patient's initial level of care or whether a change to a different level of care is appropriate, it is important to consider a constellation of factors, including the patient's overall physical condition, behaviors, affective state, cognitions, and social circumstances (see Table 5 and Table 6). Services for the treatment of eating disorders can range from intensive inpatient programs (in which general medical care is readily available), to residential and partial hospitalization

TABLE 5. **Considerations in determining an appropriate level of care**

Factors that suggest significant medical instability, which may require hospitalization for acute medical stabilization, including need for monitoring, fluid management (including intravenous fluids), electrolyte replacement, or nutritional supplementation via nasogastric tube feeding (see Table 6)

Factors that would suggest a need for inpatient psychiatric treatment (e.g., significant suicide risk, aggressive behaviors, impaired safety due to psychosis/self-harm, need for treatment over objection or involuntary treatment)

Co-occurring conditions (e.g., diabetes, substance use disorders) that would significantly affect treatment needs and require a higher level of care

Lack of response or deterioration in patient's condition in individuals receiving outpatient treatment

Extent to which the patient is able to decrease or stop eating disorder and weight control behaviors (e.g., dietary restriction, binge eating, purging, excessive exercise) without meal support or monitoring

Level of motivation to recover, including insight, cooperation with treatment, and willingness to engage in behavior change

Psychosocial context, including level of environmental and psychosocial stress and ability to access support systems

Extent to which a patient's access to a level of care is influenced by logistical factors (e.g., geographical considerations; financial or insurance considerations; access to transportation or housing; school, work, or childcare needs)

programs, to varying levels of outpatient care (in which the patient receives general medical treatment, nutritional counseling, and/or individual, group, and family psychotherapy). Characteristics of such services are described in Table 7.

As an initial treatment setting, outpatient care will be appropriate for the majority of patients, although some individuals will need initial treatment in a higher level of care. Evidence-based outpatient treatment is effective and will commonly be provided by a coordinated multidisciplinary team (Golden et al. 2015b). The processes by which care coordination occur will differ with the setting and with the expertise and responsibilities of multidisciplinary team members but should be discussed and agreed upon in advance to ensure optimal care.

Outpatient treatment has the advantage of allowing patients to remain with their families and continue to attend school or work; however, patients and their families should understand that a higher level of care may be necessary if weight control behaviors or eating disorder symptoms are worsening or if progress is not seen over 6 weeks (e.g., as evidenced by an average weight gain of 0.5–1 lb/week in individuals with AN, 50% decrease in purging behaviors for individuals with AN or BN). Thus, for individuals treated in an outpatient setting, careful monitoring is essential and includes at least weekly weight determinations done directly after the patient voids, with shoes and outerwear removed. Depending on the patient's clinical presentation and symptoms, orthostatic pulse and orthostatic blood pressure may also need to be measured on a regular basis. Additionally, in patients who purge, it is important to monitor serum electrolytes with a monitoring frequency determined by prior electrolyte values, purging frequency, and other aspects of the patient's clinical condition.

A number of factors can suggest that a higher level of care is needed, either initially or following a trial of outpatient treatment. These include low weight in relation to estimated individually determined target weight, rate of recent weight loss, medical complications of purging, evidence of medical instability (e.g., vital sign abnormalities, severe electrolyte disturbances), approaching a weight at which instability previously occurred in the patient, additional stressors that affect the patient's eating disorder behaviors, the degree of the patient's difficulties in collaborating in their care, and co-occurring psychiatric symptoms or diagnoses that suggest a need for a higher level of care or that merit inpatient admission in their own right. Insufficient weight gain or worsening eating disorder symptoms despite treatment can also suggest a need for a higher level of care. Each patient will differ in the degree to which these factors may influence decisions about the most appropriate care setting, and individuals will not necessarily move in a sequential fashion from one level on the care

TABLE 6. One or more factors supporting medical hospitalization or hospitalization on a specialized eating disorder unit

	Adults	Adolescents (12–19 years)
Heart rate	<50 bpm	<50 bpm
Orthostatic change in heart rate	Sustained increase of >30 bpm	Sustained increase of >40 bpm
Blood pressure	<90/60 mmHg	<90/45 mmHg
Orthostatic blood pressure	>20 mmHg drop in sBP	>20 mmHg drop in sBP
Glucose	<60 mg/dL	<60 mg/dL
Potassium	Hypokalemia[1]	Hypokalemia[1]
Sodium	Hyponatremia[1]	Hyponatremia[1]
Phosphate	Hypophosphatemia[1]	Hypophosphatemia[1]
Magnesium	Hypomagnesemia[1]	Hypomagnesemia[1]
Temperature	<36°C (<96.8°F)	<36°C (<96.8°F)
BMI	<15	<75% of median BMI for age and sex
Rapidity of weight change	>10% weight loss in 6 months or >20% weight loss in 1 year	>10% weight loss in 6 months or >20% weight loss in 1 year
Compensatory behaviors	Occur frequently and have either caused serious physiological consequences or not responded to treatment at lower level of care	Occur frequently and have either caused serious physiological consequences or not responded to treatment at lower level of care
ECG	Prolonged QTc >450 or other significant ECG abnormalities	Prolonged QTc >450 or other significant ECG abnormalities
Other conditions	Acute medical complications of malnutrition (e.g., seizures, syncope, cardiac failure, pancreatitis)	Acute medical complications of malnutrition (e.g., seizures, syncope, cardiac failure, pancreatitis), arrested growth and development

Note. BMI=body mass index; bpm=beats per minute; ECG=electrocardiogram; sBP=systolic blood pressure.
[1]Reference ranges for potassium, sodium, phosphate, and magnesium and numerical thresholds for values that determine hypokalemia, hyponatremia, hypophosphatemia, and hypomagnesemia depend upon the clinical laboratory.

continuum to the next. Furthermore, there is no algorithmic approach that can determine the optimal care setting with certainty. For example, individuals may have had prior experiences in a particular treatment program or level of care that will influence current decision-making. In addition, consequences of nutritional restriction in children and adolescents can contribute to negative effects on neuronal development, impairments in concentration leading to poorer educational outcomes, loss of BMD, and arrested physical growth and development (Bang et al. 2021; Hemmingsen et al. 2021; Modan-Moses et al. 2021; Workman et al. 2020). A child or adolescent with a rapid loss of weight may also become medically compromised more rapidly than an adult with a similar amount or rate of weight loss. As compared to adults, resting vital signs also differ in children, who will typically have a higher resting heart rate and lower systolic blood pressure. Children and adolescents may also be more affected by stressful family dynamics or school-related stressors, including bullying or cyberbullying. On the other hand, older patients or those with chronically low weight may be at heightened risk as compared to younger individuals with shorter illness durations because of long-term malnutrition or multiple medical comorbidities. Older patients may also have additional stressors (e.g., financial, occupational, social) or fewer psychosocial supports as compared to children and adolescents who are residing with family.

For individuals who require inpatient care, the choice of a specific program should be made based on the patient's psychiatric and medical status, the skills and abilities of local psychiatric and

TABLE 7. Characteristics of levels of care

Level of care	Specialized pediatric/medical inpatient eating disorders program	General pediatric/medical inpatient program	Specialized psychiatric inpatient eating disorders program	General psychiatric inpatient program
Unit security	Unlocked	Unlocked	Typically locked	Typically locked
Patient legal status	Voluntary or involuntary	Voluntary	Voluntary or involuntary	Voluntary or involuntary
Physician on-site 24/7	On-site 24/7	On-site 24/7	On-call or on-site 24/7	On-call or on-site 24/7
Nursing on-site 24/7	On-site 24/7	On-site 24/7	On-site 24/7	On-site 24/7
Medical monitoring	Frequent	Frequent	Frequent	Frequent
Hours of operation	24/7	24/7	24/7	24/7
Able to maintain work/school	School, in some instances	School, in some instances	School, in some instances	School, in some instances
Available interventions				
Option for IV hydration	Yes	Yes	On some units	On some units
Option for nasogastric tube feedings	Yes	Yes	On some units	On some units
Option for treatment over objection	Yes	Yes	Yes	Yes
Medical management	Yes	Yes	Consultation	Consultation
Psychiatric management	Yes	Consultation	Yes	Not eating disorder specific
Psychological management	Yes	In some instances	Yes	On some units, not eating disorder specific
Group-based therapies	Yes	No	Yes	Not eating disorder specific
Individual psychotherapies	Yes	Generally not available	Yes	Not eating disorder specific
Family psychotherapies	Yes	Generally not available	On some units	Not eating disorder specific
Meal supervision and support	All meals/day	In some instances	All meals/day	Not eating disorder specific
Milieu therapy	Yes	No	Yes	Not eating disorder specific
Nutritional management	Yes	Consultation	Yes	Consultation
Multidisciplinary team-based management	Yes	In some instances, not eating disorder specific	Yes	Not eating disorder specific

Guideline Statements and Implementation

TABLE 7. Characteristics of levels of care *(continued)*

Level of care	Residential program	Partial hospital	Intensive outpatient	Outpatient
Unit security	Unlocked	Unlocked	Unlocked	Unlocked
Patient legal status	Voluntary	Voluntary	Voluntary	Voluntary
Physician on-site 24/7	On-call 24/7	Typically not on-site full-time	Not on-site full-time	No
Nursing on-site 24/7	Typically on-site 24/7	Typically not on-site full-time	Typically not on-site full-time	No
Medical monitoring	Limited	Limited	Limited	As indicated
Hours of operation	24/7	Variable hours per day (5–12 hours) and days per week (5–7)	3–4 hours per day, 3–7 days per week	1–2 psychotherapy sessions per week with additional visits with other clinicians as indicated
Able to maintain work/school	School, in some instances	School, in some instances	Often	Yes
Available interventions				
Option for IV hydration	No	No	No	No
Option for nasogastric tube feedings	Typically not	No	No	No
Option for treatment over objection	No	No	No	No
Medical management	Limited consultation	Limited consultation	No	Outpatient, as indicated
Psychiatric management	Yes	Yes	Variable	As indicated
Psychological management	Yes	Yes	Yes	Yes
Group-based therapies	Yes	Yes	Yes	As indicated
Individual psychotherapies	Yes	Yes	Yes	Yes
Family psychotherapies	Yes	Yes	Yes	Yes
Meal supervision and support	All meals/day	2–3 meals/day	~1 meal/day	Provided by family or care partners
Milieu therapy	Yes	Yes	Yes	No
Nutritional management	Yes	Yes	Variable	As indicated
Multidisciplinary team-based management	Yes	Yes	Yes	As indicated

medical staff, and the availability of suitable programs to care for the patient's psychiatric and other medical problems. In general, however, outcomes are likely to be better when patients are treated on inpatient units staffed with experts in treating eating disorders than when treated in general medical or psychiatric inpatient settings where staff lack expertise and experience with eating disorders. Furthermore, expert eating disorders behavioral specialty programs can improve eating disorder symptomatology and restore weight in the majority of underweight patients using a multidisciplinary approach that includes supervised meals, behavioral contingency management strategies, and individual, group, and family-based treatments (Attia and Walsh 2009). Patient and program characteristics may also play a role in determining the pluses and minuses of program choice. For example, many programs will only accept voluntary patients, which can influence treatment site access and selection. Insurance-related considerations are another common source of difficulty in accessing an appropriate level of care (Guarda et al. 2018; Walker et al. 2020).

In patients of all ages, legal interventions, including involuntary hospitalization and legal guardianship, may be necessary to address the safety of treatment-reluctant patients whose medical conditions are life-threatening. In such circumstances, involuntary treatment is ethically and clinically justified only when a patient's decision-making capacity regarding appropriate treatment for their eating disorder is impaired, the risk of death or serious morbidity is high, and the likelihood of benefit from involuntary treatment outweighs the risk of harm. There is a limited amount of data on treatment outcomes with involuntary treatment of AN; however, in general, rates of mortality with long-term follow-up do not appear to differ for those who have received involuntary treatment as compared to voluntary treatment (Atti et al. 2021; Ward et al. 2015). Such findings are encouraging because involuntarily treated patients with AN have a higher severity of overall symptoms, a larger number of prior hospitalizations, a lower BMI at the time of admission, and a higher likelihood of having comorbid conditions than patients who are admitted voluntarily (Atti et al. 2021).

When shifts are made in the setting or location of care, continuity of care is essential. Transition planning requires that the care team in the new setting or locale be identified and that specific patient appointments be made. It is preferable that a specific clinician on the team be designated as the primary coordinator of care to ensure continuity and attention to important aspects of treatment.

Weight status, per se, or other physiological or behavioral markers should never be used as a sole criterion for transition to a less intensive setting. For example, patients who are physiologically stabilized on acute medical units will still require specific inpatient treatment for eating disorders if they do not meet medical, psychiatric, and behavioral criteria for less intensive levels of care and/or if no suitable, less intensive levels of care are accessible because of geographical or other reasons. Individuals with atypical AN may still be malnourished and be at risk for complications regardless of their current weight or BMI (Whitelaw et al. 2018). Assisting patients in determining and practicing appropriate food intake at a healthy weight is likely to decrease the chances of their relapsing after transitioning to a less intensive setting. If transitions between settings of care occur too frequently or after only brief periods of time, it can disrupt therapeutic relationships, sabotage patient progress, and lead to poorer outcomes.

Peer-support programs can supplement but should not replace professionally provided treatment for an eating disorder. Programs that provide peer support can reduce feelings of shame or stigma, decrease social isolation, assist with sustaining of recovery, and help families understand eating disorders. Such programs differ in their emphasis but focus on self-acceptance, improved body image, increased physical movement, and better nutrition and health. On the other hand, programs that focus on abstaining from specific food groups are nutritionally problematic and can interfere with recovery. Many patients and families are also accessing helpful information through websites, newsgroups, chat rooms, and social media. In some instances, however, the lack of professional supervision within these resources may result in unhealthy dynamics among users or in perpetration of misinformation. Thus, it is recommended that clinicians inquire about a patient's or family's use of peer- or internet-based support and openly discuss the information, ideas, and approaches to eating that have been gathered from these sources.

Anorexia Nervosa

STATEMENT 10: Medical Stabilization, Nutritional Rehabilitation, and Weight Restoration for Patients With Anorexia Nervosa

APA *recommends* (1C) that patients with anorexia nervosa who require nutritional rehabilitation and weight restoration have individualized goals set for weekly weight gain and target weight.

Implementation

Medical stabilization, nutritional rehabilitation, weight restoration, and maintenance of weight gain are critical components of treatment for AN that focus on helping the patient achieve and maintain a healthy and medically appropriate weight for their age and height. The same principles will apply to individuals with other restrictive eating disorders, including ARFID and atypical AN, and may also apply to individuals with other eating disorder diagnoses who require weight restoration. The goals of nutritional rehabilitation for seriously underweight, malnourished, or medically unstable patients are to restore medical stability (e.g., normalize vital signs, electrolytes, and fluid balance), restore weight, correct biological and psychological sequelae of malnutrition, normalize eating patterns, and achieve normal perceptions of hunger and satiety.

Nutritional rehabilitation may be achieved in a variety of settings (e.g., outpatient, day treatment program, residential, hospital) and will depend on the patient's medical and psychiatric stability. The setting where a patient is engaged in weight restoration will vary according to a number of factors, including age, severity of illness, available psychosocial support networks, and available treatment options (see Table 7). For individuals who are markedly underweight, hospital-based programs for nutritional rehabilitation should be considered. Weight restoration for adolescents and emerging adults with AN will often occur as an outpatient under the supervision of their parents/caregivers (e.g., with FBT). Outpatient weight restoration may also be appropriate for some adult patients, provided they are able to demonstrate consistent increases in weight; however, a higher level of care may be needed if weight control behaviors or eating disorder symptoms are worsening or if progress is not seen over 6 weeks (e.g., as evidenced by an average weight gain of 0.5–1 lb/week). For those in inpatient or residential settings, the weight at which it is appropriate to discharge a patient may vary in relation to the patient's individually determined target weight and will depend on the patient's ability to feed themselves, the patient's motivation and ability to participate in treatment, and the availability and adequacy of programs at a lower level of care. In general, the closer a patient is to their individually determined target weight before discharge, the less risk they will have of relapsing and being readmitted. Having patients maintain their weight for a period of time before they are discharged from inpatient or residential treatment likely decreases the risk of relapse as well.

To help patients normalize eating and weight control behaviors, most specialty inpatient and residential programs employ supervised meals and group therapies as well as some level of behavioral contingency management as part of a structured behavioral treatment protocol. With such an approach, positive reinforcements (e.g., privileges) and negative consequences (e.g., required bed rest, exercise restrictions, restrictions of off-unit privileges) are built into the program; negative consequences can then be reduced or terminated and positive reinforcements accelerated as target weights and other goals are achieved.

Renourishment should be implemented in nurturing emotional contexts. Staff should convey to patients their intention to take care of them and not let them die even when the illness prevents the patients from taking care of themselves. If the patient experiences an element of a structured treatment program as aversive, the staff should clearly communicate the rationale for programmatic protocols—that the aim is to help shape and reinforce behaviors and choices aligned with health. Ongoing staff training and peer support models may be useful to support staff members in providing empathic care. As discussed in Statement 9, compulsory treatment is ethically and clinically justified only when a patient's decision-making capacity regarding appropriate treatment for their eating disorder is impaired, the risk of death or serious morbidity is high, and the likelihood of benefit from involuntary treatment outweighs the risk of harm.

Setting individually determined target weights

Individually determined target weights should be established as part of the initial treatment plan. Typically, the target weight will be discussed explicitly with the patient, but this can require considerable sensitivity. On occasion it may be judicious to delay this discussion until the patient is less fearful of their ultimate weight. Similarly, patients differ in the extent to which they wish to be informed of their weight, with some wanting to know specific values and others wanting only to know whether they have met their weekly weight targets. In adolescents, target weight will be adjusted upward to correspond to increases in the patient's height, and it can be helpful to discuss this with them from the initiation of treatment. During a period of growth, the target weight should be reassessed every 3–6 months.

One estimate of a target weight is the weight at which reproductive physiology normalizes (e.g., restoration of normal menstruation and ovulation, restoration of normal testicular function). Typically, menses will resume at approximately 90%–95% of median BMI (Dempfle et al. 2013; Faust et al. 2013; Golden et al. 1997, 2008). This is typically about 5 lb greater than the weight at which menses ceased and corresponds to a threshold for body fat percentage of approximately 21% (Traboulsi et al. 2019). In adults with AN, a BMI of 20 can also be used as an initial guide when determining a target weight. For individuals with atypical AN, a target weight may be somewhat higher than a BMI of 20 and should be individualized based on the patient's weight history, normalization of eating patterns, and achievement of medical stability.

For adolescents and young adults, setting the individualized target weight should include assessment of the patient's premorbid height, weight, and BMI percentiles; menstrual history (in adolescents with secondary amenorrhea); and current pubertal stage (Golden et al. 2015a). Growth curves should be followed and are most useful when longitudinal data are available, given that extrapolations from cross-sectional data at one point in time can be misleading. Bone age may be accurately estimated from wrist X-rays and nomograms. In conjunction with bone measurements, mid-parental heights, assessments of skeletal frame, and Centers for Disease Control and Prevention growth charts (available at www.cdc.gov/growthcharts) may be used to accurately estimate individually appropriate ranges for "expected" weights for current age.

Setting individualized goals for caloric intake and weekly weight gain

The period of weight restoration following medical stabilization and the resumption of regular caloric intake may take several months depending on the patient's weight and nutritional status at commencement of treatment. In working to achieve target weights, the treatment plan should also establish expected rates of controlled weight gain. Clinical consensus suggests that realistic targets are 2–4 lb/week for patients in residential or inpatient programs, at least 1–3 lb/week for patients in partial hospital programs, and at least 1–2 lb/week for individuals in outpatient programs. In addition, for individuals treated in outpatient programs, a higher level of care may be necessary if weight control behaviors or eating disorder symptoms are worsening or if progress is not seen over 6 weeks of treatment (e.g., as evidenced by an average weight gain of 0.5–1 lb/week in individuals with AN; see Statement 9).

Historically, initial caloric prescriptions for patients beginning nutritional rehabilitation were conservative (e.g., 1,000 to 1,200 kcals/day) due to concern for precipitating refeeding syndrome; however, lower calorie renourishment protocols have been associated with poor weight gain (Garber et al. 2012, 2013; Golden et al. 2013) and longer hospitalizations (Garber et al. 2021; Golden et al. 2013). Many programs are now using higher initial caloric prescriptions (e.g., 1,500 to 2,000 kcal/

day) and faster rates of renourishment because the literature has not shown an association between higher caloric intake during nutritional rehabilitation and the development of refeeding syndrome when patients are under close medical monitoring with electrolyte correction (e.g., for hypophosphatemia) as needed (Garber et al. 2016, 2021; Golden et al. 2021; Redgrave et al. 2015; Society for Adolescent Health and Medicine 2014; Strandjord et al. 2015, 2016). Data from both inpatient and outpatient settings indicate that early weight gain (Wade et al. 2021) and a faster rate of weight gain (Lund et al. 2009) are associated with better outcomes, providing further support for a more robust approach to acute nutritional rehabilitation.

As weight restoration proceeds, daily caloric intake should be gradually increased, with most patients requiring between 3,000 and 4,000 kcal/day to achieve a regular rate of weight gain. Individuals with AN experience a rise in resting energy expenditure on resumption of increased daily caloric intake (Krahn et al. 1993; Obarzanek et al. 1994; Rigaud et al. 2007b; Schebendach et al. 1997), further increasing the total number of calories they require to achieve weight gain. Patients who require significantly higher caloric intakes may have a truly elevated metabolic rate or may be discarding food, vomiting, exercising frequently, or engaging in significant amounts of isometric exercise or non-exercise motor activity, such as fidgeting. In patients who report lower caloric intake, rapid weight gain may reflect the presence of hidden objects (e.g., weights) or water loading to artificially inflate weight measurements. In these circumstances, weight should be measured after voiding with the patient clothed in a gown. A urine specific gravity test may also be helpful in ascertaining whether weight was artificially inflated by excessive water intake.

Registered dietitian nutritionists will typically be involved in nutritional rehabilitation and should have sufficient training and experience in treating individuals with an eating disorder (Academy for Eating Disorders Nutrition Working Group 2021; Hackert et al. 2020). Registered dietitian nutritionists can help patients choose their own meals, provide a structured meal plan that ensures nutritional adequacy, and often establish or guide plans for caloric and dietary goals, nutrient balance (including adequate fat, protein, and carbohydrate), vitamin needs, food variety, and eating of regularly scheduled meals and snacks (Heruc et al. 2020; International Association of Eating Disorders Professionals Foundation 2017). Ongoing nutrition counseling will typically be needed as weight restoration and renourishment proceed in order to implement the eating plan and make adjustments to address challenges that arise. Registered dietitian nutritionists may also intervene directly with patients, serve as coaches to parents in family-based therapies, and consult with other members of the treatment team.

Many programs utilize a meal-based approach in which patients receive a combination of regularly scheduled and monitored meals and snacks. Calorie-dense liquid supplements can be prescribed as snacks or between meals to reach weight gain goals. It is also important to encourage patients with AN to expand their food choices because patients will typically have a severely restricted range of foods that are initially acceptable to them. In addition, many individuals will give rationalizations for restricted eating. A careful history may be needed from the patient and from collateral sources of information to identify longstanding cultural or religious practices relating to food as compared to recent restrictions in food choice with the onset of an eating disorder. It can also be challenging to distinguish between a preference to avoid specific foods, fear of eating specific foods, food intolerances, and true food allergies.

Some acute medical and psychiatric programs also use supplemental nasogastric tube (NGT) feeding for acute nutritional rehabilitation in patients who are unable to achieve their prescribed meal-based caloric intake. The decision to use NGT feeding varies with patient age, other clinical characteristics, and availability of specialized treatment programs (e.g., meal-based behavioral treatment for eating disorders); it is not necessarily indicated based solely on medical instability or severity of illness (e.g., BMI in a dangerously low range). NGT feeding can lead to an increase in weight and may be employed when patients do not otherwise consume a sufficient number of calories for weight gain, but it has little or no impact on normalizing food intake or increasing dietary or macronutrient variety (Agostino et al. 2013; Garber et al. 2016; Rigaud et al. 2007a; Robb et al.

2002). Use of NGT feeding can also be associated with complications such as nasal irritation, epistaxis, electrolyte disturbance, patient distress, and patient-initiated NGT removal (Hindley et al. 2021). Consequently, NGT feeding should be viewed as a short-term intervention with the goal of transitioning to oral intake. In addition, the potential benefits of NGT feeding need to be weighed against the possibility that a patient may develop iatrogenic complications of NGT feeding, become dependent on NGT feeding for nutritional support, use NGT feeding as a way to avoid oral intake, or become overly focused on somatic symptoms in relation to NGT feeding. When it is used, NGT feeding can be delivered continuously, overnight, or in several boluses during the day depending on the needs and preferences of the patient. In rare situations in which longer-term NGT feeding is required, feeding through surgically placed gastrostomy or jejunostomy tubes may be an alternative to nasogastric feeding (Neiderman et al. 2000). However, the use of such an approach is not preferred. Total parenteral nutrition is not recommended and should only be considered in extreme circumstances when all other options for nutritional supplementation have been attempted (Garber et al. 2016). In addition, total parenteral nutrition requires intensive medical monitoring and has an increased risk of serious complications (e.g., hepatic injury, sepsis, disseminated intravascular coagulation; Michihata et al. 2014; Weinsier and Krumdieck 1981). Frequent reassessment of the treatment plan and the patient's progress will be needed to avoid harm. In situations in which involuntary forced feeding is considered, careful thought should be given to clinical circumstances, family opinion, and relevant legal and ethical dimensions of the patient's treatment.

Physical health considerations during medical stabilization and nutritional rehabilitation

The risk of medical sequelae from acute nutritional rehabilitation in malnourished patients with AN is the most pronounced during the first week of renourishment. Weight gain results in improvement in most of the physiological complications of starvation, and the risk of medical sequelae declines over the subsequent weeks of renourishment.

Refeeding syndrome is the most serious complication and can present with a range of clinical symptoms, including rhabdomyolysis, hemolytic anemia, seizure, cardiac arrhythmias, cardiac failure or arrest, coma, and sudden death (da Silva et al. 2020; Rio et al. 2013). Hypophosphatemia that develops in the setting of acute nutritional rehabilitation (i.e., refeeding hypophosphatemia) is the hallmark biochemical marker of refeeding syndrome (Garber et al. 2016); however, the development of refeeding syndrome is rare and can be prevented by close medical monitoring (Garber et al. 2016; Golden et al. 2015a). A patient's serum levels of phosphorus, magnesium, potassium, and calcium should be determined daily until stabilized. If patients are exhibiting persistent vomiting, regular monitoring of serum potassium levels is recommended. Phosphorus, magnesium, and/or potassium supplementation should be given when indicated and, in most circumstances, can be given orally. In addition to monitoring for electrolyte abnormalities, hypoglycemia, including postprandial hypoglycemia, is often observed (Braude et al. 2020; Guinhut et al. 2021; Kinzig et al. 2007).

Initial assessments should include vital signs and food and fluid intake and output, if indicated, as well as monitoring for edema, rapid weight gain (associated primarily with fluid overload), and congestive heart failure. Typically, edema can be managed by providing patients with education and reassurance. Nevertheless, patients who misuse laxatives or diuretics are at risk of developing severe edema when these are suddenly discontinued, presumably from salt and water retention caused by elevated aldosterone levels associated with chronic dehydration. Caution should be taken with intravenous rehydration in severely malnourished patients, especially in individuals who misuse laxatives or diuretics. Any intravenous fluids should be administered at slow rates and titrated judiciously to minimize third spacing and edema.

ECGs should be performed as indicated depending on the patient's vital signs, the presence of electrolyte abnormalities, the presence of arrhythmias or QTc prolongation on prior ECGs, and other clinical factors. For children and adolescents who are severely malnourished as well as for patients with recent syncope or ECG abnormalities (e.g., prolonged QTc interval, extreme bradycardia), cardiac monitoring, especially at night, may be desirable until the patient's condition has stabilized.

GI dysmotility disorders are extremely common in individuals with eating disorders (Norris et al. 2016; Schalla and Stengel 2019; West et al. 2021). These disorders are exacerbated by or can be direct consequences of starvation and binge eating and purging behaviors. Dysmotility symptoms can also intensify during early renourishment but generally improve with weight restoration. For example, with renourishment, patients may experience abdominal pain and bloating with meals that results from the delayed gastric emptying that accompanies malnutrition. These symptoms may respond to short-term use of pro-motility agents such as metoclopramide, but monitoring is needed to detect the emergence of drug-induced parkinsonism, acute dystonia, or tardive dyskinesia. Constipation may be ameliorated with fiber laxatives, stool softeners, or other osmotic agents such as polyethylene glycol. In severe starvation or in patients with a history of laxative misuse, constipation may become severe and, rarely, progress to acute bowel obstruction. Use of stimulant laxatives such as senna products or bisacodyl is not typically recommended; however, if these medications are used, they should be closely monitored and reserved for significant constipation that is unresponsive to stool softeners, fiber laxatives, and osmotic agents.

Psychological considerations during nutritional rehabilitation

Ambivalence toward treatment focused on weight restoration is a hallmark of AN. As weight gain proceeds, resulting changes in body shape and function may be distressing and generate doubts about treatment. In addition, patients who require hospitalization usually enter care under some degree of pressure from others, which can contribute to high levels of perceived coercion. Importantly, insight and motivation for recovery typically improve with reversal of the starved state, normalization of eating and weight control behaviors, and treatment of co-occurring conditions.

Weight gain also results in improvements in psychological complications of semistarvation. Although it is by no means certain that patients' abnormal eating habits will improve simply as a function of weight gain, there is considerable evidence to suggest that other eating disorder symptoms diminish as weight is restored and maintained. For example, clinical experience indicates that with weight restoration, food choices increase, food hoarding decreases, and obsessions about food decrease in frequency and intensity, although they do not necessarily disappear. Attention, concentration, and other cognitive effects of semistarvation also improve with renourishment.

At the same time, staff should help patients deal with their concerns about weight gain and body image changes, given that these are particularly difficult adjustments for patients to make. In fact, there is general agreement among clinicians that distorted attitudes about weight and body shape are the least likely to improve with weight restoration and typically lag changes in weight and eating behavior. Thus, it is important to warn patients about the following aspects of early recovery: as they start to recover and feel their bodies getting larger, especially as they approach numbers on the scale that represent phobic weights, individuals may experience a resurgence of anxious and depressive symptoms, irritability, and sometimes suicidal thoughts. These mood symptoms, non-food-related obsessional thoughts, and compulsive behaviors, although often not eradicated, will usually decrease over several months following weight restoration if weight is maintained and restrictive eating, binge eating, or purging behaviors do not recur. If mood symptoms and non-food-related obsessions and compulsions persist, further assessment should occur to identify co-occurring disorders and implement additional treatment for any such disorders, as appropriate.

Physical activity during nutritional rehabilitation

An individual assessment of motivations, benefits, and risks of exercise should be done for each patient as part of treatment planning and be reassessed as renourishment proceeds. Treatment planning should also consider whether compulsive or driven exercise was a part of the patient's eating disorder–related behaviors (Dittmer et al. 2018; Dobinson et al. 2019). For all patients, physical activity should be adapted to the patient's food intake, energy expenditure, BMD, and cardiac function. For the severely underweight patient, exercise should always be carefully supervised and monitored; it should be restricted to no more than 1.5 hours/week or stopped if weight is not gained. Once a safe weight is achieved, the focus of an exercise program should be on gaining physical fitness as opposed to expending calories. The focus on fitness should be balanced with restoring patients' positive relationship with their bodies—helping them take back control and get pleasure from physical activities rather than feeling compelled to engage in exercise. Consequently, an exercise program should be developmentally appropriate and enjoyable and have endpoints that are not determined by time spent expending calories or by effects on weight and body shape. Weight training to promote bone health and team sports such as soccer, basketball, volleyball, or tennis are preferable to solitary activities. For competitive athletes, decisions about an individual's return to full participation in sports will require balancing health-related factors, risks of participation in the designated sport, and other factors that may influence decision-making about participation (De Souza et al. 2014; Fredericson et al. 2021; Quesnel et al. 2019).

Use of medication to support weight gain during nutritional rehabilitation

There is limited evidence for benefits of medication to support weight gain during nutritional rehabilitation. Furthermore, the clinical trial data that exist are almost entirely from studies of adults. Consequently, the decision about whether to use psychotropic medications and, if so, which medications to choose will be based on the patient's age and clinical presentation. In addition, many patients with AN are extremely reluctant to take medications, particularly ones that they know result in weight gain. These issues must be discussed empathetically and comprehensively with patients and, for children and adolescents, with their families as part of shared decision-making. The limited empirical data do not show any advantages of selective serotonin reuptake inhibitors (SSRIs) in terms of weight gain (Barbarich et al. 2004; Fassino et al. 2002; Halmi et al. 2005; Kaye et al. 2001; Ruggiero et al. 2003; Walsh et al. 2006; Yu et al. 2011); however, these medications are commonly used (Garner et al. 2016; Monge et al. 2015), are relatively well tolerated, and may be considered for those with persistent depressive, anxiety, or obsessive-compulsive symptoms. If antidepressants are considered for co-occurring disorders in adolescents and emerging adults, clinicians should attend to the boxed warnings relating to antidepressants and discuss the potential benefits and risks of antidepressant treatment with patients and families (U.S. Food and Drug Administration 2018). Of the other antidepressants, bupropion is contraindicated for use in patients with purging behaviors (e.g., laxative use, self-induced vomiting), given the increased risk of seizures observed in early clinical trials in patients with BN who received high-dose immediate-release bupropion (Horne et al. 1988; Pesola and Avasarala 2002). Medications that prolong QTc intervals, either alone or in combination with other medications, should also be used cautiously in patients with purging behaviors (Funk et al. 2018; Woosley et al. 2022). Medication such as olanzapine may be useful in selected patients to assist with weight gain; however, potential adverse effects (e.g., glucose dyscontrol, metabolic syndrome, akathisia, extrapyramidal effects) need to be considered (Attia et al. 2019). Despite the high levels of anxiety in some patients related to eating, use of a benzodiazepine as an anxiolytic agent does not appear to be beneficial (Steinglass et al. 2014) and carries a risk of misuse. Electroconvulsive therapy (ECT) has generally not been useful in individuals with AN except in treating severe co-occurring disorders, such as major depressive disorder or catatonia, for which ECT is otherwise indicated (Andersen et al. 2017; Pacilio et al. 2019; Shilton et al. 2020).

In terms of assisting with weight gain during nutritional rehabilitation, hormonal therapies (e.g., transdermal estradiol, human growth hormone) do not appear to confer any advantages, but studies have been limited (Bloch et al. 2012; Divasta et al. 2012; Faje et al. 2012; Golden et al. 2002; Gordon et al. 2002; Klibanski et al. 1995; Misra et al. 2011). Use of hormonal therapies to improve BMD is described in the "Treatments to Improve Bone Mineral Density in Patients With Anorexia Nervosa" section that follows.

Treatments to improve bone mineral density in patients with anorexia nervosa

Individuals of all genders with AN can experience a loss of BMD, typically assessed by DXA. To reduce the risk of osteopenia, osteoporosis, and bone fractures (e.g., in hips or spine), it is optimal to focus on weight restoration (El Ghoch et al. 2016). Other treatments for osteopenia or osteoporosis have limited evidence and possible risks that should be weighed against potential benefits to bone health in patients with AN. For example, oral hormone replacement therapy has sometimes been given to improve BMD in amenorrheic patients, but no good supporting evidence exists either in adults or in adolescents to demonstrate its efficacy (Bloch et al. 2012; Divasta et al. 2012, 2014; Faje et al. 2012; Golden et al. 2002; Gordon et al. 2002; Hornberger et al. 2021; Klibanski et al. 1995; Misra et al. 2011; Strokosch et al. 2006). In addition, the American College of Obstetricians and Gynecologists (2018) recommends against the use of combined oral contraceptive pills in individuals with eating disorders when the sole purpose is treatment of amenorrhea. Furthermore, estrogen can contribute to the fusion of the epiphyses and should not be administered before growth is completed (Allen et al. 2021; Mosekilde et al. 2013; Shim 2015). Use of estrogen also requires intermittent administration of progesterone, and the occurrence of monthly bleeding may provide false reassurance about the adequacy of the patient's weight, even when additional weight gain is needed. For older adolescents (bone age ≥15 years) who are unable to gain and sustain weight gain and have a BMD Z-score <-2.0, one might consider the application of 17β estradiol patch (100 μg twice weekly) with cyclic oral progesterone for 10–12 days every month (Misra et al. 2011). Bisphosphonates may be considered in adults with osteoporosis, particularly when there is a history of fractures, but should be used cautiously in women of childbearing age due to possible teratogenic risk. In addition, use of these medications can be associated with negative effects, including the infrequent occurrence of osteonecrosis of the jaw. Data on the use of denosumab are minimal and limited to case reports (Anand and Mehler 2019; Jamieson and Pelosi 2016).

If dietary calcium intake is inadequate or if vitamin D levels are <30 ng/mL, calcium and/or vitamin D supplementation should be considered, although there is no evidence that such supplementation normalizes BMD. In addition, with calcium, increasing ingestion via food is preferable to supplementation. If supplementation is used, limiting doses of calcium to 1,200 mg/day may minimize the risks of use, which include an increased possibility of renal stones or cardiovascular calcification. If vitamin D levels are low (<30 ng/mL), recommended treatment includes repletion of vitamin D stores with ergocalciferol 50,000 IU once a week for 6–8 weeks, accompanied by a maintenance dose of 1,000–2,000 IU vitamin D_2 or D_3 daily (Golden et al. 2014; Institute of Medicine 2011b). Weight training has also been suggested to promote bone health after weight restoration has been achieved; however, information on the benefit of this approach is limited.

Weight maintenance/stabilization

There are limited data to support specific relapse prevention-focused interventions and a lack of consensus within the field on how to define relapse, remission, and recovery. Nevertheless, existing data suggest that patients are at the highest risk for relapse during the first year following treatment and elevated risk extending into the second year (Berends et al. 2018). The duration of treatment will vary with the treatment approach and individual patient needs; however, continuation of treatment after patients have completed weight restoration is important to support maintenance of weight gain and help prevent the return to prior patterns of eating behavior during this high-risk period. Following intensive treatment and successful weight restoration, adequate caloric intake but lower dietary variety and fat intake may be associated with higher relapse risk and may signal a need for additional nutritional rehabilitation (Schebendach et al. 2008, 2012). The available evidence does not suggest a specific benefit for use of SSRIs in addition to CBT in reducing relapse risk in patients whose weight has been restored (Walsh et al. 2006), although these medications may be used to treat co-occurring disorders during the weight maintenance phase of treatment.

STATEMENT 11: Psychotherapy in Adults With Anorexia Nervosa

APA *recommends* **(1B)** that adults with anorexia nervosa be treated with an eating disorder–focused psychotherapy, which should include normalizing eating and weight control behaviors, restoring weight, and addressing psychological aspects of the disorder (e.g., fear of weight gain, body image disturbance).

Implementation

Psychotherapy is appropriate as an initial intervention in all age groups. It is also appropriate in the weight restoration and relapse prevention stages of treatment. In addition to a focus on normalizing eating and weight control behaviors and restoring weight, psychotherapy should include consideration of other factors, such as body image normalization and eating-related cognitions.

During acute renourishment, it is beneficial to provide patients with AN with individual psychotherapeutic management that provides empathic understanding, explanations, praise for positive efforts, coaching, support, encouragement, and other positive behavioral reinforcement. Initiation of an eating disorder–focused psychotherapy is also integral to the treatment of AN, although the timing should be individualized based on the patient's medical stability and readiness to engage in psychotherapy. For example, with severely malnourished patients, attempts to conduct formal psychotherapy may be ineffective. The goals of psychotherapeutic interventions include helping patients with AN 1) discuss their experience of their illness; 2) cooperate with their nutritional and physical rehabilitation; 3) change the behaviors and dysfunctional attitudes (e.g., cognitive distortions) related to their eating disorder; 4) identify developmental, familial, and cultural antecedents of their illness; 5) address comorbid psychopathology, psychological conflicts, adaptive benefits of symptoms, and family or cultural factors that reinforce or maintain eating disorder behaviors; 6) improve their coping skills and their interpersonal and social functioning; 7) resume age-appropriate life roles (e.g., school, work, relationships); and 8) address other quality of life concerns. During weight maintenance phases of treatment, psychotherapy can also help patients address residual concerns relating to body image, body shape, and weight acceptance. During this phase, psychotherapy can help patients identify areas for continued progress (e.g., further normalization of eating and exercise behavior, resumption of functional life roles) and learn how to avoid or minimize the risk of relapse, including specific concerns about possible abuse, neglect, or developmental traumas and approaches to better cope with salient developmental and other important life issues or stressors in the future. Patients' responses to the therapist, including transference, can be influenced by the characteristics of the therapist (e.g., age, gender, ethnicity, body size), and it is important to attend to these issues, if present. In addition, clinicians need to attend to their countertransference reactions to patients with a chronic eating disorder, which often include beleaguerment, demoralization, and excessive need to change the patient. Consultation with other clinicians can be helpful in managing these responses.

In terms of specific psychotherapies, research studies often describe these interventions as distinct, but features of psychotherapies are often shared (see Table 8), and there is frequent overlap of the psychotherapeutic interventions used in clinical practice.

Some approaches, such as FBT, emphasize a time-limited model of treatment; however, for individuals with AN of long duration, psychotherapeutic treatment is frequently required for at least 1 year and may take many years. For patients whose illness is resistant to treatment, more extensive psychotherapeutic measures may be undertaken to engage and help motivate patients, because patients can experience substantial remission even after many years of illness (Dobrescu et al. 2020; Eddy et al. 2017; Eielsen et al. 2021).

Among the psychotherapies that have been examined, those with modest efficacy in treating AN in adults include CBT (eating focused and broadly focused), focal psychodynamic psychotherapy (FPT), interpersonal therapy (IPT), Maudsley Model of Anorexia Nervosa Treatment for Adults

(MANTRA), and Specialist Supportive Clinical Management (SSCM). Experienced Carers Helping Others (ECHO) is aimed at supporting carers of patients with AN but can also contribute to improved outcomes. Psychotherapies that appear to be effective in treating adolescents and emerging adults are discussed in Statement 12.

Cognitive-behavioral therapy for anorexia nervosa

Many of the earlier clinical trials investigating CBT for AN were based on guidelines provided by Garner et al. (1997). The essence of CBT for AN is the focus on changing weight-related behaviors and beliefs about food and weight through challenging cognitive distortions (F.A. Carter et al. 2011; J.C. Carter et al. 2009; Dalle Grave et al. 2013a; Garner et al. 1997; McIntosh et al. 2005; Pike et al. 2003). This includes challenging rationalizations that reinforce restrictive eating, either positively (e.g., that restriction and weight loss behaviors are "healthy" or indicate control or mastery of one's behavior) or negatively (e.g., that eating a single serving of caloric foods will lead to catastrophic weight gain or loss of control of eating). For the latter, reinforcement can include reductions in fears of weight gain, but it may also include more complex meanings, such as, for example, avoidance of psychosexual development and intimate interpersonal relationships. Treatment initially emphasizes building the therapeutic alliance and enhancing motivation for treatment, in part, through the establishment of this personalized formulation and the recognition by the therapist of the ways in which weight loss behaviors are reinforced. CBT includes a direct focus on eating disorder symptoms and an examination of core beliefs (i.e., schemas) and themes, such as self-control and perfectionism. Typically, during the session, the clinician and the patient check the patient's weight together, and the patient's self-monitoring records and homework from the prior session are reviewed. There is an initial focus on establishing a pattern of regular eating and then increasing the size and variety of meals and snacks. Strategies to reduce purging behaviors are also addressed, if relevant. An experimental model of change is incorporated throughout treatment to test out new behaviors as a way to acquire new information to challenge beliefs around the value of weight loss. The therapeutic relationship can also serve as a model of how the individual interacts with others, which then permits dysfunctional core beliefs to be identified and cognitive distortions challenged, with the goal of decreasing social avoidance and increasing interpersonal intimacy. Psychoeducation is embedded throughout treatment with a focus on the negative consequences of starvation on physical health as well as psychosocial effects, such as increasing rigidity and social avoidance.

Enhanced cognitive-behavioral therapy

Enhanced CBT (CBT-E) refers to a more formalized, manual-based version of CBT for eating disorders that is transdiagnostic in its emphasis and designed to disrupt the cognitive-behavioral processes that maintain the psychopathology of an eating disorder (Fairburn 2008; Fairburn et al. 2003). Treatment is guided by an individualized formulation of the patient's difficulties, constructed at the beginning of therapy, and is then revised as indicated. Although CBT-E was initially designed for adult outpatients with eating disorders (Fairburn 2008; Fairburn et al. 2003), it was subsequently adapted for use with adolescents (Dalle Grave and Calugi 2020; Dalle Grave et al. 2013b) and with patients who require a higher level of care (Dalle Grave et al. 2013a). For patients who are underweight and require weight restoration, CBT-E is delivered in about 40 sessions over 40 weeks, whereas for those who are not significantly underweight, CBT-E is usually delivered in 20 sessions over 20 weeks. Irrespective of treatment length, there is an initial emphasis on addressing the eating disorder psychopathology (i.e., focused CBT-E), with the addition of modules that address one or more "external" maintaining mechanisms (e.g., clinical perfectionism, low self-esteem, marked interpersonal difficulties) when these features are severe and are disrupting treatment progress (i.e., broad CBT-E; Cooper and Fairburn 2011).

The initial focus of treatment with CBT-E is on gaining a mutual understanding of the patient's eating disorder and engaging the patient in treatment. There is also an emphasis on personalized

TABLE 8. **Components of psychotherapies for the treatment of anorexia nervosa**

	CBT-AN	CBT-E	FPT	SSCM	MANTRA	ECHO	AFT	FBT
In-session weighing	X	X		X	X			X
Individualized case formulation	X	X	X		X		X	X
Motivational phase of treatment	X	X	X		X	X	X	
Focus on interpersonal issues/emotional expression	X	X	X	X	X	X	X	(indirectly)
Monitoring of symptoms, including eating	X	X	X	X	X	X	X	X
Examining association of symptoms/eating with cognitions	X	X						
Focus on building activities/passions to minimize overconcern with weight/body shape	X	X		If raised by patient		X		X
Use of an experimental mindset to change attitudes and behaviors	X	X			X			X
Parent-facilitated meal supervision						X		X

Note. AFT=adolescent-focused individual therapy; CBT-AN=cognitive-behavioral therapy for anorexia nervosa; CBT-E=enhanced cognitive-behavioral therapy for eating disorders; ECHO=Experienced Carers Helping Others; FBT=family-based therapy/treatment; FPT=focal psychodynamic psychotherapy; MANTRA=Maudsley Model of Anorexia Nervosa Treatment for Adults; SSCM=specialist supportive clinical management.

education that addresses regular eating and concerns about weight. The goal of CBT-E is that patients themselves decide to regain weight rather than having this decision imposed on them. The next phase of treatment addresses weight regain and the processes that maintain the patient's eating disorder. Usually, this involves addressing concerns about body shape, eating, and extreme dietary restraint and enhancing the patient's ability to deal with day-to-day events and mood changes. Every 4 weeks, a session is partly dedicated to reviewing the progress and obstacles and planning for subsequent treatment. The final phase of CBT-E is dedicated to helping the patient become accomplished at maintaining their weight.

Focal psychodynamic psychotherapy

FPT, as compared to CBT and related approaches, places a greater focus on interpersonal relationships and insight rather than on cognitions and behavior (Friederich et al. 2019; Wild et al. 2009; Zipfel et al. 2014). At the beginning of treatment, a structured operationalized psychodynamic diagnosis is formulated that delineates the patient's experience with AN (including its physical and psychological impact), patterns of interpersonal relationships, major conflicts (e.g., intimacy, attachment, self-worth, control), and strengths as well as difficulties in ego-functioning (Cierpka et al. 2007; Schneider et al. 2008). FPT typically consists of 40–50 sessions that initially occur twice weekly and then weekly for 6 months or so, tapering to less frequent sessions with the possibility of follow-up sessions after therapy ends. The first phase of treatment, which lasts 4–6 weeks, involves establishing a therapeutic alliance, building self-esteem, and helping patients verbalize their inner experience. This includes identifying pro-anorexia beliefs that reinforce eating behaviors and other beliefs, values, and feelings related to the patient's sense of self. Before every treatment session, the patient's weight is measured by an independent person who reports the weight to the treating clinician; however, during this initial phase, the therapist avoids a premature focus on weight gain. During the second phase of treatment, increased emphasis is placed on weight and the associations between eating behavior and feelings, particularly with regard to interpersonal relationships. There is also a focus on underlying psychological themes and conflicts that appear connected to the patient's eating behaviors. The final phase of FPT is aimed at helping the patient transfer insights gained from the therapy experience to everyday life, to anticipate and discuss approaches for handling relapse, and to discuss feelings and relationship themes that emerge in relation to therapy termination.

Specialist Supportive Clinical Management

SSCM typically consists of 20 or more weekly sessions and helps individuals with AN to address symptoms of eating disorders within a reassuring context (McIntosh et al. 2006). As part of SSCM, elements of clinical management include education about the disorder; ongoing monitoring of symptoms, including in-session weighing; and tracking of eating and related weight loss behaviors. This follows a detailed history in which the patient and therapist agree on target symptoms to monitor. Review of these target symptoms at each session is aimed at helping patients identify links between symptoms and eating behaviors. Physical health is also monitored, and psychoeducation is provided about healthy eating and consequences of sustained symptoms and weight loss. Once target symptoms are discussed and addressed, the remainder of the session focuses on content chosen by the patient. As treatment progresses and symptoms improve, more of the session is focused on the patient's chosen content.

Maudsley Model of Anorexia Nervosa Treatment for Adults

The model underpinning MANTRA proposes that AN has four essential interacting elements (Byrne et al. 2017; Schmidt et al. 2012, 2015, 2016). These include an information-processing style characterized by rigidity in thinking and an attention to detail that may miss the larger context; impairments in social and emotional functioning that interfere with the formation of friendships and development of intimacy; the occurrence of starvation that intensifies these problems and the belief that AN is a solution to them; and an interpersonal network that may inadvertently accommodate or enable behaviors and/or may exhibit high levels of expressed emotion. Treatment with MANTRA is based on flexible delivery of the MANTRA workbook modules and typically consists of 20 sessions. In an initial phase of treatment, the therapist employs strategies of motivational interviewing and develops an individualized case formulation in collaboration with the patient that explores the costs and perceived benefits of AN. Results from neuropsychological testing are incorporated into this formulation to illustrate how an individual's style of information processing may impact functioning. This joint conceptualization is presented in the form of a letter and diagram to the patient. In the change phase, problems with social and emotional functioning are addressed, with behavioral experiments that address these impairments. For those with chronic AN, there is a module on identity development outside of AN.

Experienced Carers Helping Others

In ECHO, carers or psychology students with minimal prior clinical experience provide telephone coaching support to caregivers who are currently managing their child's AN on an outpatient basis (Hodsoll et al. 2017; Magill et al. 2016; Salerno et al. 2016). The support is based on a published book (Treasure et al. 2007) and uses strategies of motivational interviewing. ECHO is based on the interpersonal maintenance model of AN. According to this model, individuals may inadvertently reinforce behaviors of AN via carer behavioral patterns such as accommodation, enabling, and expressed emotion (e.g., criticism, overprotection). Thus, helping carers develop skills that reduce such behaviors may improve the outcomes of adolescent AN. Parents perform a self-assessment in which they determine if they are engaging in any behaviors that might inadvertently reinforce eating disorder behaviors. Parents then develop personalized strategies to address these behaviors. In addition, parents are taught behavior change principles and cognitive styles associated with eating disorders to help them better understand their child's experience.

STATEMENT 12: Family-Based Treatment in Adolescents and Emerging Adults With Anorexia Nervosa

APA *recommends* **(1B)** that adolescents and emerging adults with anorexia nervosa who have an involved caregiver be treated with eating disorder–focused family-based treatment, which should include caregiver education aimed at normalizing eating and weight control behaviors and restoring weight.

Implementation

FBTs that include caregiver education are effective as a treatment for AN in adolescents. They are less well studied but likely to also be helpful in emerging adults ages 18–26 years of age. Family-based interventions are not limited to family members, per se, but could involve other non-family caregivers with whom the patient resides.

FBT for AN is a manual-based approach that focuses on the effects of severe weight loss as being central to the core psychology of AN (Le Grange 1999; Lock and Le Grange 2013). The focus of FBT is to enlist parents as experts on parenting their child and have them oversee and take responsibility for nourishing the child or adolescent back to an optimal weight range. One of the central tenets of FBT is to take a non-ideological stance to disorder onset. One purpose of this emphasis is to alleviate the significant blame that parents with a child with AN have historically experienced. The therapist acts as knowledge expert and facilitator; however, it is the parents who come up with solutions on how best to nourish their child. This process is facilitated by an in-session family meal to which parents bring a meal that they would feed their child. This in-session meal is a crucial part of therapy and allows the therapist to observe the approaches the parents use. For example, if parents' own eating behaviors are abnormal or restrictive, this can influence their approach to engaging their child in eating. Through gentle questioning, the therapist helps the parents arrive at strategies that would be most optimal for the child within their family context. For example, cultural beliefs and practices related to eating may be explored and used in developing the parents' approach to the child's eating.

At the beginning of each FBT session, the therapist weighs the patient and discusses the patient's current concerns, emotions, and thoughts. These data are presented to the family for use in discussion about strategies at home that are working or need to be enhanced. Other elements of the treatment can include providing information about nutrition and addressing eating-related cognitions and body image normalization. As treatment progresses to Phase 2, more responsibility for independent eating is given to the adolescent and, in Phase 3, the transition to typical adolescent development is discussed. When the patient has not gained sufficient weight after 1 month of treatment, a variation of FBT has been tested in which parents engage in more in-session family meals with more intense parental coaching (Lock et al. 2015b). These sessions are intended to help the parents engage in problem-solving to address barriers to implementation and reinvigorate the family around the severity of illness and the need for intense support and supervision. Treatment may also need to be adapted for higher levels of care (Freizinger et al. 2021; Halvorsen et al. 2018; Huryk et al. 2021; Spettigue et al. 2019).

The treatment may need to be adapted depending on the developmental needs of the patient. For example, with emerging adults as compared to young teens, it can be helpful to have the young adult give input on the type of mealtime support they prefer and to specifically consider age-appropriate situations such as attending college, beginning work, or living apart from family (Chen et al. 2016; Dimitropoulos et al. 2018; Gorrell et al. 2019). Adaptations or augmentative approaches to FBT have been developed (Gorrell et al. 2019; Lock et al. 2015b; Richards et al. 2018), including multifamily formats (Baudinet et al. 2021; Eisler et al. 2016) and a parent-focused format in which the therapist meets primarily with the parent and patient monitoring is conducted by another member of the treatment team (Le Grange et al. 2016).

For some adolescents and emerging adults, FBT may not be readily accessible due to geographical or other constraints. Small studies and significant experience during the COVID-19 pandemic suggest that FBT can be delivered using a telehealth platform to make care more readily available (Andersen et al. 2017; Hellner et al. 2021; Matheson et al. 2020). For other patients, FBT may not be feasible due to patient or family preferences or a lack of involved family members or non-family caregivers who are able and willing to engage in treatment. Other individuals may have been treated with FBT without achieving a significant response. In such circumstances, other family or individual approaches to psychotherapy may be helpful.

Adolescent-focused therapy (AFT), originally referred to as ego-oriented individual therapy, is aimed at helping patients identify their emotions and learn to tolerate negative affective states (Fitzpatrick et al. 2010; Lock et al. 2010; Robin et al. 1999). The therapist interprets the patient's behavior and emotions to help them distinguish emotional states from bodily needs, such as eating. Other themes in treatment include a focus on separation and individuation. Psychoeducation related to nutrition and effects of malnutrition is incorporated into treatment. Weight restoration occurs during the 32–40 sessions of AFT; however, in contrast to FBT, in which the parents or other carers assume responsibility for the patient's eating, AFT encourages the patient to change their own eating behaviors and gain weight. Meetings with family can occur with AFT but are used to assess parental functioning and provide updates on progress. In studies of this approach, AFT had comparable outcomes to FBT at the end of treatment but was less likely to lead to full remission of AN at follow-up assessments. In terms of other psychotherapies, systemic family therapy has been studied (Agras et al. 2014), as has CBT-E (Le Grange et al. 2020); both appear to have outcomes comparable to those of FBT.

Bulimia Nervosa

STATEMENT 13: Cognitive-Behavioral Therapy and Serotonin Reuptake Inhibitor Treatment for Adults With Bulimia Nervosa

APA *recommends* (1C) that adults with bulimia nervosa be treated with eating disorder–focused cognitive-behavioral therapy and that a serotonin reuptake inhibitor (e.g., 60 mg fluoxetine daily) also be prescribed, either initially or if there is minimal or no response to psychotherapy alone by 6 weeks of treatment.

Implementation

The aims of treatment for patients with BN are to 1) reduce and, where possible, eliminate binge eating and purging; 2) treat physical complications of BN; 3) enhance patients' motivation to cooperate in the restoration of healthy eating patterns and participate in treatment; 4) provide education regarding healthy nutrition and eating patterns; 5) encourage increased food variety and minimization of food restriction; 6) encourage healthy but not compulsive exercise patterns; 7) help patients reassess and change core dysfunctional thoughts, attitudes, motives, conflicts, and feelings related to the eating disorder; 8) address other themes that may underlie eating disorder behaviors (e.g., developmental issues, identity formation, body image concerns, self-esteem, sexual and aggressive difficulties, affect regulation, sex role expectations, family dysfunction, coping styles, problem solving); 9) treat associated psychiatric conditions, including deficits in mood and impulse regulation, self-esteem, and behavior; 10) enlist family support and provide family counseling and therapy when appropriate; and 11) prevent relapse.

Nutritional intake is important to assess for all patients with BN regardless of their body weight or BMI because normal weight does not imply appropriate nutritional intake. Adequate nutritional intake and structured eating can prevent cravings and promote satiety. In addition, helping the patient develop a structured meal plan can aid in reducing episodes of dietary restriction and urges to binge and purge. Nutritional interventions also are valuable in increasing the variety of foods eaten. Nutrition counseling with a registered dietitian nutritionist is often needed to implement the eating plan and to make adjustments to address challenges that arise (e.g., co-occurring physical health conditions, frequent work-related schedule changes or travel) (Academy for Eating Disorders Nutrition Working Group 2021; Hackert et al. 2020).

Several approaches are possible for the initial treatment of an adult with BN. Many patients show a reduction in binge eating and purging behaviors with CBT alone; however, the combination of CBT plus high-dose fluoxetine (60 mg/day) is associated with somewhat better responses than fluoxetine alone (Goldbloom et al. 1997). For this reason, initial treatment could also include a combination of CBT and an SSRI (e.g., high-dose fluoxetine). Decisions about initiating treatment with psychotherapy alone as compared to combination treatment will depend on factors such as symptom severity, co-occurring disorders, and patient preferences. Nevertheless, the best long-term outcomes occur when the initial treatment response is relatively rapid (Mitchell et al. 1993). Thus, if there is minimal or no response to psychotherapy alone by 6 weeks of treatment, addition of an SSRI will typically be warranted. Antidepressants or other psychopharmacological agents may also be used to treat specific co-occurring disorders, such as depressive, anxiety, obsessive-compulsive, or posttraumatic stress disorders.

Pharmacotherapy in bulimia nervosa

Of the SSRIs, fluoxetine is preferred as a medication choice because it has the greatest strength of research evidence showing efficacy in BN (Fluoxetine Bulimia Nervosa Collaborative Study Group 1992; Goldstein et al. 1995; Kanerva et al. 1995; Mitchell et al. 2001), independent of effects on mood (Goldstein et al. 1999). Fluoxetine has also shown benefit in a small study of individuals who had not responded to psychotherapy or had relapsed after receiving psychotherapy (Walsh et al. 2000). If symptoms do not appear to be responding to medication, it is important to assess whether the patient has taken the medication and whether medication absorption has been affected by the timing of ingestion relative to episodes of vomiting. In addition, studies show that high doses of fluoxetine (e.g., 60 mg/day) are more effective in treatment of BN than doses of 20 mg/day (Fluoxetine Bulimia Nervosa Collaborative Study Group 1992). In terms of monitoring for side effects during treatment, insomnia, nausea, and asthenia were seen in 25%–33% of patients at the dosage of 60 mg/day, and sexual side effects were common in the multicenter fluoxetine trials (Fluoxetine Bulimia Nervosa Collaborative Study Group 1992; Goldstein et al. 1995; Kanerva et al. 1995; Mitchell et al. 2001). The potential for drug-drug interactions should also be considered because fluoxetine acts as a potent inhibitor of the CYP2D6 isoenzyme and can inhibit the CYP2C19 isoenzyme at high doses (Lexicomp 2021). For patients who have responded to fluoxetine, limited evidence supports continuing fluoxetine for relapse prevention (Romano et al. 2002), typically for a minimum of 9 months.

Other SSRI antidepressants may be used in patients who are unable to tolerate fluoxetine or who prefer a different medication; however, evidence is limited on the effects of other SSRIs or other antidepressants in BN. Nevertheless, given the need for higher doses of fluoxetine for clinical effects in BN, doses at the high end of the usual dosing range are warranted if another SSRI antidepressant is used. Caution is needed with citalopram, however, because its use has been associated with QTc prolongation at doses >40 mg/day (Lexicomp 2021). In addition, clinicians should attend to the boxed warning relating to antidepressants in young adults and discuss the potential benefits and risks of antidepressant treatment with patients if such medications are to be prescribed (U.S. Food and Drug Administration 2018). Of the other antidepressants, bupropion is contraindicated for use in individuals with BN, given the increased risk of seizures observed in individuals with bulimia in early clinical trials of high-dose immediate-release bupropion (Horne et al. 1988; Pesola and Avasarala 2002). For individuals who are receiving treatment with lithium, caution is needed to avoid toxicity due to dehydration in patients who vomit or purge using laxatives.

Psychotherapy in bulimia nervosa

Cognitive-behavioral therapy

When used for the treatment of BN, CBT is commonly delivered in an individual format, but group CBT is also effective (Agras et al. 1989; Chen et al. 2003; Davis et al. 1999; Fairburn et al. 1993; Freeman et al. 1988; Ghaderi 2006; Grenon et al. 2017; Griffiths et al. 1994, 1996; Leitenberg et al. 1988; Nevonen and Broberg 2006; Sundgot-Borgen et al. 2002; Treasure et al. 1994). CBT for BN has typically been delivered based on the CBT-E approach of Fairburn and colleagues (Fairburn 2008). In the majority of clinical trials, participants received 14–21 sessions of CBT, each lasting 40–60 minutes, although a few studies used a shortened course of 8 weeks of treatment and one trial included up to 60 sessions of treatment. CBT was sometimes given weekly and sometimes given at a frequency of twice weekly at the start of treatment, decreasing to weekly for the majority of treatment and tapering to once every 2 weeks at the end of treatment. In clinical practice, some patients may require more than 21 sessions of CBT for full treatment response, and some may require a longer period with less frequent sessions to maintain treatment gains.

CBT-E for BN consists of several phases (Fairburn 2008). In the first phase, patients are given education about BN and the effects of dieting, self-induced vomiting, or purging as forms of weight control. They are also taught to engage in self-monitoring of symptoms, asked to identify situations that trigger binge eating or purging, and encouraged to establish a regular eating pattern of at least three adequate meals each day. Behavioral approaches may also be incorporated, such as eating more slowly and mindfully. The development of the therapeutic alliance is another essential ingredient of this initial treatment phase. The second phase of treatment includes a greater emphasis on problem solving, development of more constructive coping strategies, and a focus on cognitive restructuring, including identification of dysfunctional beliefs related to food, eating, weight, and body shape that perpetuate bulimic behaviors. When indicated, other dysfunctional beliefs can also be examined related to issues such as interpersonal relationships, low self-esteem, and perfectionism. After identifying these negative thoughts, patients learn to evaluate them and counter these thoughts with alternatives. Graded behavioral tasks may also be used to test these alternatives. Patients are encouraged to expand their food variety and incorporate foods into their diet that may have previously been avoided. The final phase of treatment is aimed at maintaining progress from the earlier phases of treatment and developing skills and self-efficacy to reduce risks of relapse.

Other psychotherapies

Evidence for psychotherapies other than CBT is more limited; however, some clinicians incorporate other psychotherapeutic approaches, such as interpersonal or psychodynamic therapies, into treatment (Agras et al. 2000; Murphy et al. 2012; Poulsen et al. 2014; Stefini et al. 2017; Thackwray et al. 1993). Although most psychotherapeutic interventions have been studied in relatively brief, time-limited trials, individuals who have not responded to an initial course of treatment may benefit from a change in the treatment approach or a longer duration of treatment. Longer treatment durations may also be needed for individuals with more severe symptoms or those with co-occurring disorders. Other therapeutic modifications can also be considered, depending on the patient's age, family situation, cognitive and psychological development, psychodynamic issues, cognitive style, comorbid psychopathology, and preferences. For example, integrative cognitive-affective therapy showed efficacy compared to CBT-E in one study and emphasizes the interplay between emotion regulation, interpersonal relationships, cognitive patterns, adaptive coping, and self-directed behaviors, including bulimic symptoms (Wonderlich et al. 2014). Dialectical behavior therapy (DBT) skills training has not been well studied in patients with BN but may be useful in individuals with other psychiatric disorders for which DBT would be indicated (Ben-Porath et al. 2020; Kröger et al. 2010; Safer et al. 2001).

Other interventions in bulimia nervosa

Depending on patient preference or the availability of other treatments for BN, guided self-help (GSH) could be used as an initial treatment. GSH involves a manual-based approach (Fairburn 2013), with guidance provided by a health professional who does not specialize in eating disorders (e.g., mental health professional, primary care clinician) or a peer support specialist. Notably, the addition of coaching and guidance appears to be important in improving outcomes over self-help alone (Bailer et al. 2004). The use of Web-based approaches has shown feasibility for delivery of GSH, and telehealth approaches to CBT also are feasible and show good efficacy (Mitchell et al. 2008; Zerwas et al. 2017). If there is minimal or no response to GSH by 4 weeks of treatment, referral to a health professional with experience in treating eating disorders is indicated.

STATEMENT 14: Family-Based Treatment in Adolescents and Emerging Adults With Bulimia Nervosa

APA *suggests* (2C) that adolescents and emerging adults with bulimia nervosa who have an involved caregiver be treated with eating disorder–focused family-based treatment.

Implementation

As in the treatment of AN, FBT has evidence of benefits in the treatment of BN for adolescents or emerging adults who reside with family or other carers who are able to participate in treatment (Le Grange et al. 2007, 2015; Schmidt et al. 2007).

FBT for BN is similar to the manual-based approach for AN (Le Grange 1999; Lock and Le Grange 2013) as described in Statement 12; however, it focuses on addressing the secrecy, shame, and dysfunctional eating patterns of BN by developing a more collaborative relationship with parents or other carers. As a result, adolescents and emerging adults are assisted in resuming a typical developmental trajectory.

In some instances, FBT may not be feasible due to geographical or access constraints, patient or family preferences, or a lack of involved family members or non-family caregivers who are able and willing to engage in treatment. In other circumstances, a patient may have been treated with FBT without a complete response. For such individuals, CBT either adapted for adolescents or using a therapist-led GSH approach can be considered (Dalle Grave et al. 2021; Le Grange et al. 2015; Schmidt et al. 2007).

Use of fluoxetine or other SSRIs has not been well studied to treat BN in adolescents, although emerging adults have been included in some of the adult research studies. If antidepressant treatment is otherwise indicated for a co-occurring disorder, fluoxetine has been well studied in treatment of depression and anxiety disorders in this age group (Cipriani et al. 2016; Wang et al. 2017) and has the best evidence for efficacy in BN in adults (see Statement 13). If an antidepressant is considered, however, the potential benefits and risks of treatment should be discussed with patients (and parents or guardians as appropriate), and clinicians should attend to the boxed warnings relating to antidepressants in adolescents and young adults (U.S. Food and Drug Administration 2018).

Binge-Eating Disorder

STATEMENT 15: Psychotherapy in Patients With Binge-Eating Disorder

APA *recommends* (1C) that patients with binge-eating disorder be treated with eating disorder–focused cognitive-behavioral therapy or interpersonal therapy in either individual or group formats.

Implementation

Psychotherapy with CBT or IPT shows short- and long-term benefits for BED outcomes (Hilbert et al. 2019). The aims of treatment for patients with BED are to 1) reduce and, where possible, eliminate binge eating; 2) enhance patients' motivation to participate in treatment and cooperate in the restoration of healthy eating patterns; 3) provide education regarding healthy nutrition and eating patterns; 4) encourage increased food variety and minimization of food restriction, if present; 5) help patients reassess and change core dysfunctional thoughts, attitudes, motives, conflicts, and feelings related to binge eating; 6) address other themes that may underlie eating disorder behaviors (e.g., developmental issues, identity formation, body image concerns, self-esteem, sexual and aggressive difficulties, affect regulation, sex role expectations, family dysfunction, coping styles, problem solving); 7) treat associated psychiatric conditions, including deficits in mood and impulse regulation, self-esteem, and behavior; 8) enlist family support and provide family counseling and therapy when appropriate; and 9) prevent relapse.

Nutritional intake is important to assess for all patients with BED regardless of their body weight or BMI, because normal weight does not imply appropriate nutritional intake. Dietary restriction or weight suppression can be present but may not be identified without a detailed nutritional history. In addition, restrictive interventions aimed at weight loss may fuel binge eating. A history of food insecurity has also been associated with disordered eating, including binge eating (Hazzard et al. 2020). Helping the patient develop a structured meal plan with adequate nutritional intake can reduce dietary restriction, if present, and can also promote satiety, prevent craving, and reduce urges to binge eat. Nutritional interventions also are valuable in increasing the variety of foods eaten. Nutrition counseling with a registered dietitian nutritionist is often needed to implement the eating plan and make adjustments to address challenges that arise (e.g., co-occurring physical health conditions, frequent work-related schedule changes or travel) (Academy for Eating Disorders Nutrition Working Group 2021; Hackert et al. 2020).

Cognitive-behavioral therapy

Of psychotherapies for BED, CBT is the most widely studied (Agras and Bohon 2021). There is substantial evidence supporting its efficacy for behavioral and psychological symptoms, whether it is delivered in an individual or a group format. In individual formats, studies of CBT for BED typically include 16–22 weekly sessions of 40–60 minutes, whereas in group formats 8–19 sessions lasting 60–150 minutes have been used. Groups vary in size from 6 to 12 members, and sessions are usually weekly, although session frequency may be reduced toward the end of treatment. In clinical trials, CBT has been based on one of several manuals (Fairburn 1995; Fairburn et al. 1993; Telch et al. 1990), but the general approach involves three phases of treatment. In the initial phase, there is a focus on establishing the therapeutic relationship, enhancing motivation, providing education on BED, and encouraging a pattern of eating three balanced meals with regular snacks. Patients are also taught to monitor food intake, binge-eating episodes, and associated thoughts and feelings. In the second phase, precipitants to binge-eating episodes are identified, and individuals are taught to recognize and challenge dysfunctional cognitions that trigger binge eating or that relate to eating, body weight, or body shape. Problem-solving approaches and more effective coping behaviors are developed. At this phase, some researchers also incorporate identification of negative schemas that contribute to cognitive distortions, add practice with stress management techniques, or address issues such as body image or self-esteem. The third phase focuses on maintaining improvements and strategies to prevent relapse, such as proactively planning for handling of situations that present a high risk for binge eating.

Effects of Web-based CBT and CBT-based GSH are modest in reducing binge eating, but these modalities can be used as an initial approach, particularly if other BED treatments are not readily accessible (Agras and Bohon 2021; Carrard et al. 2011; Grilo et al. 2005a, 2013; Loeb et al. 2000; Wagner et al. 2016). However, if these approaches are not associated with improvement, referral for more specialized treatment is indicated.

Interpersonal psychotherapy

IPT also appears to be effective in reducing binge eating (Karam et al. 2019; Wilfley et al. 1993, 2002). Studies of individual IPT used 19 sessions of 50–60 minutes over 24 weeks, with 3 sessions in the initial 2 weeks, weekly sessions for 12 weeks, and 4 sessions every 2 weeks. With group IPT, studies included 20 weekly sessions of 90 minutes each, 3 individual sessions (pre-treatment, mid-treatment, and post-treatment), and weekly personalized feedback in writing.

In IPT, treatment begins with a detailed evaluation of past and current symptoms and linkages to the patient's interpersonal and social context. From this assessment, which takes approximately 4–7 sessions, the psychotherapist develops an interpersonal case formulation, discusses and negotiates the formulation with the patient, collaboratively develops treatment goals, and provides psychoeducation about the diagnosis and treatment approaches. Treatment goals are typically aimed at addressing one of four problem areas: grief, interpersonal role disputes, role transitions, and/or interpersonal deficits. In the second phase of treatment, which consists of approximately 8–10 sessions, the psychotherapist focuses on ways in which binge-eating behaviors are related to current interpersonal situations. The psychotherapist uses these experiences to help the patient make changes in the targeted interpersonal problem area. The final phase of treatment focuses on termination and helps the patient plan ways to maintain gains and cope with interpersonal issues in the future.

STATEMENT 16: Medications in Adults With Binge-Eating Disorder

APA *suggests* (2C) that adults with binge-eating disorder who prefer medication or have not responded to psychotherapy alone be treated with either an antidepressant medication or lisdexamfetamine.

Implementation

Psychotherapy, either CBT or IPT, is recommended for the treatment of BED. However, some adults with BED may prefer medication to psychotherapy, whereas other individuals will not respond to psychotherapy alone or will have moderate to severe BED that may benefit from adjunctive pharmacotherapy. In such circumstances, two approaches to medication therapy for BED can be considered: an antidepressant medication or lisdexamfetamine.

Although CBT alone is generally associated with greater effects than antidepressant medications alone in the treatment of BED (Devlin et al. 2005, 2007; Grilo et al. 2005b, 2012b; Ricca et al. 2001), antidepressant therapy has been shown to be beneficial in reducing binge eating, independent of whether a co-occurring depressive or anxiety disorder is present (Guerdjikova et al. 2008; Hudson et al. 1998; Leombruni et al. 2008; Pearlstein et al. 2003). In addition, many individuals with BED will have a co-occurring disorder that would warrant antidepressant treatment (Devlin et al. 2005). Based on the available research evidence, there is insufficient information to recommend one antidepressant or class of antidepressants over another. Consequently, selection of an antidepressant is usually made through shared decision-making based on tolerability, side effect profile, and potential for drug-drug interactions. For this reason, tricyclic antidepressants and monoamine oxidase inhibitors are less likely to be used than other antidepressant medications. In addition, for patients who have purging behaviors or a history of purging behaviors, bupropion is contraindicated given the increased risk of seizures observed in individuals with BN in early clinical trials of high-dose immediate-release bupropion (Horne et al. 1988; Pesola and Avasarala 2002). If patients have concerns about weight gain with antidepressants, studies typically do not show changes of weight in either direction when individuals with BED receive treatment with an antidepressant.

Lisdexamfetamine has also been associated with modest short-term effects in BED (Guerdjikova et al. 2016; McElroy et al. 2015b, 2016a, 2016b, 2017). In addition, continued treatment with lisdexamfetamine was associated with less risk of relapse than when lisdexamfetamine was discontinued (Hudson et al. 2017). However, lisdexamfetamine has primarily been studied in obese patients in primary care settings, and its benefits in other patients with BED are unclear. When used in individuals with BED, the initial dosage is 30 mg once daily in the morning, with increases in dosage of 20 mg/week to a therapeutic dosage of 50–70 mg once daily (Guerdjikova et al. 2016; McElroy et al. 2015b, 2016a, 2016b, 2017). No dosage adjustments appear to be needed for individuals with hepatic dysfunction, although drug-drug interactions can occur with other medications that are metabolized through CYP2D6 hepatic enzymes (Lexicomp 2021; Takeda Pharmaceuticals et al. 2021). For individuals with renal impairment, lower dosages are indicated (i.e., 50 mg/day maximum dosage for glomerular filtration rate [GFR] 15 to <30 mL/minute/1.73 m^2; 30 mg/day maximum dosage for GFR <15 mL/minute/1.73 m^2 or in end-stage renal disease requiring hemodialysis) (Lexicomp 2021; Takeda Pharmaceuticals et al. 2021). Common side effects of lisdexamfetamine include insomnia, reduced appetite, upper abdominal pain, and xerostomia; however, these effects are typically well-tolerated with comparable rates of study withdrawal with lisdexamfetamine as with placebo (Guerdjikova et al. 2016; Lexicomp 2021; McElroy et al. 2015b, 2016a; Takeda Pharmaceuticals et al. 2021). Nevertheless, as with other stimulant medication, lisdexamfetamine treatment can be associated with modest decreases in weight and with increases in heart rate, blood pressure, anxiety, or jitteriness. Caution is needed if it is used in individuals with hypertension or cardiac disease, and more frequent monitoring of vital signs may be warranted. Individuals with psychotic symptoms or bipolar disorder or those who have risk factors for these conditions may experience a worsening of symptoms with stimulant treatment. The possibility of stimulant misuse or dependence should also be considered before deciding on treatment with lisdexamfetamine as well as during treatment.

Topiramate, either alone or in combination with CBT, has also been studied in individuals with BED and obesity (Claudino et al. 2007; McElroy et al. 2003, 2007b; Nourredine et al. 2021). Although topiramate treatment was associated with reductions in binge eating, attrition in these randomized trials was high, and adverse effects were more common in participants who received topiramate as compared to placebo. Cognitive dysfunction is commonly reported with topiramate, even at relatively low doses (Lexicomp 2021). Other adverse effects include increased risks of hyperchloremic metabolic acidosis, nephrolithiasis, and ocular problems (Lexicomp 2021). Dosage adjustment may be needed in geriatric patients and in individuals with renal or hepatic impairment. For individuals with childbearing potential, use of effective contraception is important; in utero exposure to topiramate has been associated with an increased risk in offspring of oral clefts or of being small for gestational age (Lexicomp 2021).

Areas for Further Research

As with any psychiatric disorder, there are multiple aspects of eating disorders that would benefit from further research (Hart and Wade 2020; Obeid et al. 2020; van Furth et al. 2016). These include research topics such as the following:

Prevention, Screening, and Assessment

- Determine whether identification of an eating disorder using routine or targeted screening is associated with benefits on patient-oriented outcomes
- Determine whether patient characteristics and symptoms can be used to identify patterns of disordered eating that would warrant early intervention to prevent onset of an eating disorder
- Identify risk factors for development of an eating disorder that could be used in defining subgroups of individuals who warrant prospective screening or could benefit from preventive interventions
- Identify population-based approaches to preventive interventions (e.g., address impact of social media on eating disorder development; Chung et al. 2021)
- Validate existing rating scales for screening, assessment, and session-by-session treatment change in the major types of eating disorders (e.g., AN, BN, BED, ARFID, other specified feeding and eating disorders [OSFED]) and among a broad range of ages, genders, cultures, languages, symptom patterns (e.g., focusing on eating, body shape, muscularity, driven exercise), and settings (e.g., primary care, specialty care)
- Determine whether additional screening, assessment, or longitudinal rating scales need to be developed to ensure validity and reliability in the major types of eating disorders (e.g., AN, BN, BED, ARFID, OSFED) among a broad range of ages, genders, cultures, languages, symptom patterns (e.g., focusing on eating, body shape, muscularity, driven exercise), and settings (e.g., primary care, specialty care)
- Determine whether useful clinical assessment measures might be developed based on NIMH's Research Domain Criteria (RDoC) frameworks (Monteleone et al. 2020; Schaefer and Steinglass 2021; Wildes and Marcus 2015) for measures such as appetitive signaling, anxiety related to social processes, reward learning, and reward prediction errors related to eating and thinness

Treatment Planning

- Determine ways to optimize short- and long-term patient outcomes, including recovery, using factors and approaches such as
  A. Early identification and intervention
  B. "Stepped-care" approaches, which start with less intensive treatment and shift to more intensive interventions, as needed, to achieve recovery
  C. Telehealth (individual, group, and family)
  D. Remote physiological monitoring
  E. Large-scale data analytics and predictive algorithms

F. Self-help and GSH approaches, including groups, manual-based approaches, or computer-based programs (including Web-based, phone applications, chat bots, and other modalities)

G. Family/caregiver interventions, including support groups and psychoeducation

H. Involving certified peer support specialists as part of the multidisciplinary team

I. Augmenting treatment with other psychosocial therapies (e.g., creative art therapies, cognitive remediation therapy) or complementary therapies

J. Modifying treatment to improve physical health and address co-occurring health conditions, including substance-related and addictive disorders and other psychiatric disorders

K. Modifying treatment to address significant symptoms such as suicidal ideas and behaviors, obsessions and compulsions, and perfectionism

L. Modifying treatment to address attachment-related issues or traumatic experiences, including adverse childhood experiences

M. Developing new treatments to target key processes in eating disorders (e.g., satiety, hunger, energy expenditure, cognitive rigidity, self-efficacy, body dissatisfaction, self-image disturbances)

N. Developing treatments to address transdiagnostic processes involved with eating disorders and with common co-occurring conditions

- Identify clinical indicators, biomarkers, and other factors that can help in individualizing treatment selection, frequency, and duration to achieve optimal patient outcomes
- Identify clinical indicators, biomarkers, and other factors that can help in determining an optimal sequence of treatments if an initial therapeutic modality is not associated with response or recovery
- Identify approaches to individualizing treatment selection and delivery to optimize outcomes for individuals of different ages, developmental stages, sexes, genders, races, ethnicities, and cultural groups, among other individual facets
- Identify optimal approaches to treatment of individuals with a longstanding eating disorder as compared to individuals with a more recent onset of symptoms
- Obtain additional evidence on novel or existing psychotherapies (e.g., DBT, mindfulness, acceptance and commitment therapy, mentalization-based therapy) in treatment of eating disorders
- Obtain additional evidence on novel or existing pharmacotherapies in the treatment of eating disorders
- Conduct studies on the comparative effectiveness of psychotherapies and other interventions in treating eating disorders
- Identify optimal approaches to providing multidisciplinary team–based care of eating disorders
- Determine the circumstances in which "bundled" treatment programs are appropriate to use, including the elements of these programs that enhance patient outcomes
- Identify optimal dietary and nutritional interventions for each of the eating disorders, including the ways in which these interventions may need to be adjusted to specific patient needs, symptom severity, or clinical progress
- Identify clinical considerations in assessment and monitoring as well as optimal approaches to providing treatment to individuals with an eating disorder who wish to become pregnant, are pregnant, or are breastfeeding.
- Determine which factors can be used in selecting an optimal treatment setting
- Determine optimal monitoring frequencies and approaches to detect treatment-related benefits and side effects
- Identify optimal approaches to preventing relapse once remission from an eating disorder has been achieved
- Develop "step-down" approaches to care to reduce relapse and avoid discontinuities in care
- Identify the treatment elements and approaches that are viewed as most and least helpful by individuals who have recovered from an eating disorder

- Identify methods that will allow information from mobile technologies, wearable technology, and large-scale data analytics to inform assessment, treatment, and future research
- Identify approaches to redesigning workflows and models of care delivery to improve the use of best practices and reduce inequities in the care of individuals with an eating disorder
- Determine the ways in which health system factors and treatment delivery characteristics influence patient outcomes

Anorexia Nervosa

- Determine approaches to maximize patient engagement, increase motivation for change, and facilitate treatment retention for individuals with AN
- Identify optimal nutritional approaches to weight restoration, including targeted meal-based interventions aimed at normalizing food choice, intake, dietary variety, and macronutrient content (e.g., percent fat intake)
- Determine whether supplemental approaches to feeding (e.g., NGT feeding) are indicated in AN, and if so, the optimal approaches and circumstances in which supplemental feeding can improve outcomes as compared to meal-based approaches
- Determine whether specific interventions (e.g., exposure with response prevention, mindfulness) can be used to address specific symptoms or concerns (e.g., anxiety about eating, body image disturbance)
- Identify predictive factors that distinguish between individuals who respond more quickly to treatment and those who have longer illness courses, with the aim of developing new treatment approaches for individuals with severe and enduring AN
- Determine the circumstances under which specific medications (e.g., olanzapine, antidepressants) may be useful in an individual with AN
- Determine whether there is a role for exercise in the treatment of individuals with AN and, if so, the optimal type, amount, and timing of exercise recommendations
- Identify specific approaches for maintaining weight and behavioral gains and reducing relapse risk in AN once weight restoration is achieved
- Determine ways in which treatments for AN and monitoring for medical sequelae of AN may need to be adjusted for older adults
- Determine optimal approaches for treating co-occurring disorders in an individual with AN, including whether such treatments should occur simultaneously or sequentially
- Determine optimal approaches for minimizing symptoms associated with renourishment (e.g., GI dysmotility, edema, electrolyte abnormalities, cardiac effects)
- Determine optimal approaches to prevent, identify, and treat short- and long-term medical sequelae of AN, including individual characteristics (e.g., age, gender, race, ethnicity, co-occurring conditions, family history) that can affect development of these sequelae.
- Determine the physiological and other factors that contribute to low BMD in AN, approaches to addressing BMD, and gender-associated differences in physiology and treatment of low BMD
- Determine the ways in which individuals with AN experience inequity in assessment, treatment, and outcomes due to factors such as age, gender, sexual orientation, race, ethnicity, culture, weight, body size, social determinants, and insurance status, so that these health inequities can be ameliorated

Bulimia Nervosa

- Determine whether fluoxetine or other SSRIs are effective in adolescents and emerging adults with BN

- Determine optimal approaches to treating individuals with BN who have multiple co-occurring conditions or whose diagnosis has shifted from AN-binge/purge subtype to BN
- Determine the ways in which individuals with BN experience inequity in assessment, treatment, and outcomes due to factors such as age, gender, sexual orientation, race, ethnicity, culture, weight, body size, social determinants, and insurance status so that these health inequities can be ameliorated

Binge-Eating Disorder

- Determine optimal psychotherapeutic and pharmacological approaches to treating adolescents and emerging adults with BED
- Determine whether optimal treatment approaches for individuals with BED differ in individuals who are obese as compared to those who are not obese
- Determine whether specific treatments for obesity (e.g., diet approaches, surgical approaches) are associated with a different profile of benefits and harms when used in individuals with BED
- Determine the ways in which individuals with BED experience inequity in assessment, treatment, and outcomes due to factors such as age, gender, sexual orientation, race, ethnicity, culture, weight, body size, social determinants, and insurance status so that these health inequities can be ameliorated

Avoidant/Restrictive Food Intake Disorder

- Determine optimal approaches for screening, assessment, and evaluating session-by-session treatment change in individuals with ARFID among a broad range of ages, genders, cultures, languages, and symptom patterns
- Validate potential subtypes of ARFID including their patterns of signs and symptoms as well as their natural history
- Determine optimal approaches to treating individuals with ARFID, expanding on work with parent-based approaches (Shimshoni and Lebowitz 2020) and CBT (Thomas et al. 2020, 2021) as well as developing new approaches to treatment
- Identify variations in ARFID presentation across the lifespan and whether adjustments in treatment are needed for individuals in different age groups

Other Specified Feeding and Eating Disorders

- Determine optimal approaches to treating individuals with night eating syndrome
- Determine the optimal approach to setting target weights for individuals with atypical AN
- Determine ways in which treatment for atypical AN may need to differ from treatment of AN
- Determine modifications in treatment that may be needed for individuals who have had a shift in diagnosis (e.g., from the restricting subtype to the binge/purge subtype of AN, from the binge/purge subtype of AN to BN).
- Determine the ways in which individuals with other eating and feeding disorders experience inequity in assessment, treatment, and outcomes due to factors such as age, gender, sexual orientation, race, ethnicity, culture, weight, body size, social determinants, and insurance status so that these health inequities can be ameliorated

Ethical Issues in Eating Disorder Assessment and Treatment

- Determine the optimal approaches to assess patients' capacity to accept or decline treatment in eating disorders, particularly restrictive eating disorders
- Identify circumstances under which compulsory or coercive treatment of an eating disorder may be ethically justifiable
- Determine the outcomes of compulsory or coercive treatment of an eating disorder (e.g., hospitalization, NGT feeding) as compared to declining treatment or receiving voluntary treatment
- Identify optimal approaches to providing palliative care to individuals with severe and enduring AN
- Determine optimal approaches (e.g., verbal communications, electronic information sharing via patient portals or open notes) for involving family in treatment while also protecting the privacy and confidentiality of adolescents and emerging adults
- Identify ways in which social media influences eating disorder symptoms and treatment engagement
- Determine whether specific policy recommendations, regulatory requirements, or adjustments to social media algorithms can reduce the deleterious effects of social media on individuals who have an eating disorder
- Develop methods to ensure that screening occurs in all patients undergoing a psychiatric evaluation and that diagnostic assessments are conducted in all patients reporting symptoms consistent with disordered eating, because there is no current evidence supporting ethnic or racial differences in the prevalence and presentation of eating disorders
- Identify ways eating disorder risks, assessment, treatment, and outcomes are affected by biases and discrimination (by society and by health care professionals) related to factors such as age, gender, sexual orientation, race, ethnicity, culture, weight, body size, and social determinants
- Identify effective approaches to reducing and eliminating health disparities due to bias and discrimination in the assessment and treatment of individuals with an eating disorder
- Determine whether specific policy recommendations, regulatory requirements, or health care service delivery interventions can reduce disparities in patients' access to care based on factors such as age, gender, sexual orientation, race, ethnicity, culture, weight, body size, and social determinants as well as insurance status and geographical location

Study Design Considerations

In addition to these specific topics that would benefit from additional research, our ability to draw clinically meaningful conclusions from research would be augmented by improvements in the design of studies. These include

- Improve the generalizability of study populations
- Enhance study recruitment approaches and use a priori specification of analyses to obtain data on treatment effects in subgroups that have been underrepresented in prior research (e.g., inpatients; older individuals; individuals with multiple psychiatric or physical health conditions; individuals with severe and/or persistent illness; diverse samples of individuals in terms of gender, sexual orientation, race, ethnicity, culture, weight, body size, and social determinants)
- Develop approaches to data collection and transparent reporting of sociodemographic factors to facilitate pooling of data from multiple studies and permit assessment of treatment effects in subgroups that have been underrepresented in previous research

- Standardize collection of key data elements and outcome variables as well as information on patient characteristics that are important to risk adjustment of outcomes (e.g., BMI at admission, illness duration, age of illness onset, co-occurring conditions)
- Provide detailed information on processes used for random assignment and masking or blinding to treatment condition
- Report data separately for each diagnostic group in studies that use transdiagnostic samples
- Augment self-report observations with direct measurements of outcome, insofar as possible
- Ensure that sample sizes in clinical studies are adequate to achieve statistical power
- Ensure that studies report data in a consistent fashion with pre-specification of outcomes of interest
- When observations are missing, use appropriate data analytic approaches and perform sensitivity analyses, when indicated, to determine effects of missing data
- Identify instruments for measuring eating disorder symptoms that are efficient and accurate in measuring key outcomes for AN, BN, BED, and other eating disorders and foster standardized and consistent use of such instruments across studies
- Identify standardized approaches for collecting information about factors that ultimately may be useful in individualizing treatment selection (e.g., biomarkers, family history, symptom history, treatment history, and personality traits)
- Ensure that studies identify the magnitude of change in scale scores that would constitute a clinically meaningful difference
- Increase collection of data on patient-centered outcomes (e.g., quality of life, social functioning, physical health, recovery)
- Develop consensus definitions of response, remission, and recovery that can be applied consistently across studies
- Ensure that studies of new treatments, technologies, delivery system modifications, or clinical decision support systems include specific attention to health equitability in implementation methods
- Develop mechanisms such as registries for systematic collection of information on program outcomes as a complement to collecting clinical trial data
- Improve systematic collection of information on harms, including in studies of psychotherapies
- Ensure that studies assess longer-term treatment (e.g., at least 1 year) and long-term follow-up assessments (e.g., 3–5 years) to identify possible long-term harms and patterns of relapse after treatment completion

Additional Resources on Eating Disorders

Internet Resources

Academy for Eating Disorders	www.aedweb.org/home
Academy of Nutrition and Dietetics	www.eatright.org
American Academy of Child and Adolescent Psychiatry	www.aacap.org
American Academy of Pediatrics	www.aap.org
American Psychiatric Association	www.psychiatry.org/patients-families/eating-disorders
American Psychological Association	www.apa.org/topics/eating-disorders
Australia and New Zealand Academy for Eating Disorders	www.anzaed.org.au
Behavioral Health Nutrition Dietetic Practice Group of the Academy of Nutrition and Dietetics	www.bhndpg.org
Centers for Disease Control and Prevention (growth charts)	www.cdc.gov/growthcharts/charts.htm
Eating Disorder Registered Dietitians and Professionals	edrdpro.com
Families Empowered And Supporting Treatment for Eating Disorders	www.feast-ed.org
International Association of Eating Disorders Professionals Foundation	www.iaedp.com
National Alliance for Eating Disorders	www.allianceforeatingdisorders.com
National Association of Anorexia Nervosa and Associated Disorders	anad.org
National Eating Disorders Association	www.nationaleatingdisorders.org
National Institute of Mental Health	www.nimh.nih.gov/health/topics/eating-disorders
Society for Adolescent Health and Medicine	www.adolescenthealth.org

Books for Health Care Professionals

Agras WS, Apple RF: *Overcoming Eating Disorders: A Cognitive-Behavioral Treatment for Bulimia Nervosa and Binge-Eating Disorder*, 2nd Edition. New York, Oxford University Press, 2008 (therapist workbook)

Becker CB, Farrell NR, Waller G: *Exposure Therapy for Eating Disorders* (ABCT Clinical Practice Series). New York, Oxford University Press, 2019

Brownell KD, Walsh BT (eds): *Eating Disorders and Obesity: A Comprehensive Handbook*, 3rd Edition. New York, Guilford, 2018

Dancyger I, Fornari V (eds): *Evidence Based Treatments for Eating Disorders: Children, Adolescents and Adults*, 2nd Edition. New York, Nova Science Press, 2014

Lock J (ed): *Pocket Guide for the Assessment and Treatment of Eating Disorders*. Washington, DC, American Psychiatric Publishing, 2019

Lock J: *Adolescent-Focused Therapy for Anorexia Nervosa: A Developmental Approach*. New York, Guilford, 2020

Lock J, Le Grange D: *Treatment Manual for Anorexia Nervosa: A Family Based Approach*, 2nd Edition. New York, Guilford, 2015

Thomas JJ, Eddy KT: *Cognitive-Behavioral Therapy for Avoidant/Restrictive Food Intake Disorder: Children, Adolescents, and Adults*. Cambridge, UK, Cambridge University Press, 2019

Walsh RT, Attia E, Glasofer DR, Sysko R (eds): *Handbook of Assessment and Treatment of Eating Disorders*. Washington, DC, American Psychiatric Publishing, 2016

Westmoreland P (ed): *Tipping the Scales: Ethical and Legal Dilemmas in Managing Severe Eating Disorders*. Washington, DC, American Psychiatric Publishing, 2021

Wonderlich SA, Peterson CB, Smith TL: *Integrative Cognitive-Affective Therapy for Bulimia Nervosa: A Treatment Manual*. New York, Guilford, 2015

Books for Patients and Families

Agras WS, Apple RF: *Overcoming Your Eating Disorder Guided Self-Help Workbook: A Cognitive-Behavioral Therapy Approach for Bulimia Nervosa and Binge-Eating Disorder* (Treatments That Work). New York, Oxford University Press, 2007 (client workbook)

Andersen AE, Cohn L, Holbrook T: *Making Weight: Men's Conflicts With Food, Weight, Shape and Appearance*. Carlsbad, CA, Gürze Books, 2000

Arnold C: *Decoding Anorexia: How Breakthroughs in Science Offer Hope for Eating Disorders*, 1st Edition. New York, Routledge, 2013

Bays JC: Mindful Eating: *A Guide to Rediscovering a Healthy and Joyful Relationship with Food*, Revised Edition. Boulder, CO, Shambhala, 2017

Bryant-Waugh R: *ARFID Avoidant Restrictive Food Intake Disorder: A Guide for Parents and Carers*. London, UK, Routledge, 2020

Bulik CM, Taylor N: *Runaway Eating: The 8-Point Plan to Conquer Adult Food and Weight Obsessions*. New York, Rodale Books, 2005

Cash TF: *The Body Image Workbook* (A New Harbinger Self-Help Workbook). Oakland, CA, New Harbinger, 2008

Crosbie C, Sterling W: *How to Nourish Your Child Through an Eating Disorder: A Simple, Plate-by-Plate Approach to Rebuilding a Healthy Relationship with Food*. New York, The Experiment, 2018

Dalle Grave R, el Khazen C: *Cognitive Behaviour Therapy for Eating Disorders in Young People: A Parents' Guide*. London, UK, Routledge, 2022

Fairburn C: *Overcoming Binge Eating: The Proven Program to Learn Why You Binge and How You Can Stop*, 2nd Edition. New York, Guilford, 2013

Ganci M, Atkins L: *Unpack Your Eating Disorder: The Journey to Recovery for Adolescents in Treatment for Anorexia Nervosa and Atypical Anorexia Nervosa*. Australia, LM Publishing, 2019

Gaudiani J: Sick Enough: *A Guide to the Medical Complications of Eating Disorders*. New York, Routledge, 2019

Goodman LJ, Villapiano M: *Eating Disorders: The Journey to Recovery Workbook*. New York, Brunner-Routledge, 2018

Harrison C: Anti-Diet: *Reclaim Your Time, Money, Well-Being, and Happiness Through Intuitive Eating*. New York, Little, Brown Spark, 2019

Liu A: Restoring *Our Bodies, Reclaiming Our Lives: Guidance and Reflection on Recovery from Eating Disorders*. Boston, MA, Trumpeter, 2011

Lock J, Le Grange D: *Help Your Teenager Beat an Eating Disorder*. New York, Guilford, 2015

Mulheim L: *When Your Teen Has an Eating Disorder: Practical Strategies to Help Your Teen Recover from Anorexia, Bulimia and Binge Eating*. Oakland, CA, New Harbinger Publications, 2018 (also available in Spanish)

Norton C: *Feeding Your Anorexic Adolescent*. Nutripress, 2014

Schaefer J, Rutledge T: *Life Without Ed: How One Woman Declared Independence from Her Eating Disorder and How You Can Too*. New York, McGraw Hill, 2004

Schmidt, U, Startup, H, Treasure J: *A Cognitive-Interpersonal Therapy Workbook for Anorexia Nervosa for People With Anorexia Nervosa*. New York, Routledge, 2018

Schmidt U, Treasure J, Alexander J: *Getting Better Bit(e) by Bit(e): A Survival Kit for Sufferers of Bulimia Nervosa and Binge Eating Disorder*, 2nd Edition. New York, Routledge, 2016

Thomas JJ, Becker KR, Eddy KT: *The Picky Eater's Recovery Book*. Cambridge, UK, Cambridge University Press, 2021

Treasure J, Smith G, Crane A: *Skills-based Caring for a Loved One with an Eating Disorder: The New Maudsley Method*, 2nd Edition. London, Routledge, 2017

Tribole E, Resch E, Tylka T: *The Intuitive Eating Workbook: Ten Principles for Nourishing a Healthy Relationship With Food*. Oakland, CA, New Harbinger, 2017

Walsh BT, Attia E, Glasofer DR: *Eating Disorders: What Everyone Needs to Know*. New York, Oxford, 2020

Walsh BT, Glasofer DR: *If Your Adolescent Has an Eating Disorder: An Essential Resource for Parents*. New York, Oxford, 2020

Zucker NL: *Off the C.U.F.F.: A Parent Skills Book for the Management of Disordered Eating*. Independently published, 2020

Guideline Development Process

This guideline was developed using a process intended to meet standards of the Institute of Medicine (2011a) (now known as the National Academy of Medicine). The process is fully described in a document available on the APA Web site at: www.psychiatry.org/psychiatrists/practice/clinical-practice-guidelines/guideline-development-process.

Management of Potential Conflicts of Interest

Members of the Guideline Writing Group (GWG) are required to disclose all potential conflicts of interest before appointment, before and during guideline development, and on publication. If any potential conflicts are found or disclosed during the guideline development process, the member must recuse himself or herself from any related discussion and voting on a related recommendation. The members of both the GWG and the Systematic Review Group (SRG) reported no conflicts of interest. The "Disclosures" section includes more detailed disclosure information for each GWG and SRG member involved in the guideline's development.

Guideline Writing Group Composition

The GWG was initially composed of four psychiatrists with general research and clinical expertise (R.B., J.E., M.J.T., A.S.). This non-topic-specific group was intended to provide diverse and balanced views on the guideline topic to minimize potential bias. Three psychiatrists (E.A., A.G., V.F.), one psychologist (N.Z.), one adolescent pediatrician (N.G.), one internist (M.M.), and one dietitian (L.M.) were added to provide subject matter expertise in eating disorders. Two fellows (B.U., M.R.) were involved in the guideline development process, and an additional member (K.P.) provided input on quality measure considerations. The vice-chair of the GWG (L.J.F.) provided methodological expertise on such topics as appraising the strength of research evidence. The GWG was also diverse and balanced with respect to other characteristics, such as geographical location and demographic background. F.E.A.S.T. and Mental Health America reviewed the draft and provided perspective from patients, families, and other care partners.

Systematic Review Methodology

This guideline is based on a systematic search of available research evidence conducted by APA staff, extraction of detailed information on included studies by Dr. Evidence (Santa Monica, CA) using the DOC Data 2.0 software platform, and network meta-analyses conducted by Heno Analytics (Vancouver, BC, Canada). The systematic search of available research evidence used MEDLINE (PubMed), Cochrane Library, and PsycINFO databases, with specific search terms and limits as described in Appendix B. Results covered the period from the start of each database to July 15, 2019, and were limited to English-language and human-only studies that were clinical trials, observational studies, systematic reviews, or meta-analyses. Case reports, comments, editorials, and letters were excluded. Updated searches were conducted using the same criteria for the period from January 1, 2019, to October 1, 2021, to ensure that more recent evidence was incorporated into the guideline. Four reviewers (L.J.F., S.-H.H., J.Y., and T.C.) screened the results of the initial search, with each abstract and title screened by two reviewers according to APA's general screening criteria: RCT, systematic review or meta-analysis, or observational study with a sample of at least 50 individuals; human; study of the effects of a specific intervention or psychiatric disorder or symptoms. If discrepancies were noted among reviewers' ratings, an additional opinion was given by a third individual and consensus was achieved among the reviewers. Abstracts identified using this approach were then reviewed by one individual (S.-H.H.), with verification by a second reviewer (L.J.F.) to determine whether they met eligibility criteria as defined by the PICOT elements (see Appendix B). For the updated search, abstracts were screened in the same fashion by two reviewers (L.J.F. and S.-H.H.) with discrepancies resolved by discussion and consensus among the reviewers. If the publication characteristics were not clear from the initial title and abstract review, full text review occurred.

Studies were included if participants were ≥10 years of age and diagnosed with an eating disorder (AN, BN, BED, night eating syndrome, ARFID) with diagnosis as defined by DSM-III, DSM-III-R, DSM-IV, DSM-IV-TR, DSM-5 (Section II or Section III), or ICD-10, as applicable. Interventions of interest included psychotherapies, pharmacotherapies, and other interventions. For AN, approaches to refeeding and bone density preservation were also included. Comparator conditions included active interventions, placebo, treatment as usual, waiting list controls, or general psychiatric management. Multiple outcomes were included related to key eating disorder findings, functioning, quality of life, adverse effects, and study withdrawal rates, among others (see Appendix B). Studies were excluded if the eating disorder of interest did not account for at least 75% of the total sample. Other exclusion criteria included small sample size ($N<20$ for randomized controlled trials [RCTs], $N<50$ for non-randomized clinical trials or observational studies), lack of a comparator group, or short treatment duration (<10 days for refeeding studies or < 8 weeks for other studies). Citations to registry links, abstracts, and proceedings were not included unless also published in a peer-reviewed journal because they did not include sufficient information to evaluate the risk of bias of the study.

For each trial identified for inclusion from the search, detailed information was extracted by Dr. Evidence (Santa Monica, CA) using the DOC Data 2.0 software platform. Dr. Evidence processes included verifications and quality checks on data extraction. In addition to specific information about each reported outcome, extracted information included citation; study design; treatment arms (including doses, sample sizes); co-intervention, if applicable; trial duration and follow-up duration, if applicable; country; setting; funding source; sample characteristics (e.g., mean age, percent nonwhite, percent female, percent with co-occurring condition); and rates of attrition, among other data elements. Summary tables (see Appendices E and H) include specific details for each study identified for inclusion from the literature search. Factors relevant to risk of bias were also identified for each RCT that contributed to a guideline statement. Risk of bias was determined using the Cochrane Risk of Bias 2.0 tool (Sterne et al. 2019) by one reviewer (J.M.) and verified by an additional reviewer (S.-H.H. or L.J.F.). Risk of bias ratings are included in summary tables (see Appendix E), with specific factors contributing to the risk of bias for each study shown in Appendix F (McGuinness and Higgins 2020). Extracted data on outcomes were used in network meta-analyses (conducted by Heno Analytics; Vancouver, BC, Canada).

Available guidelines from other organizations were also reviewed (see Appendix G) (American College of Obstetricians and Gynecologists 2018; Catalan Agency for Health Technology Assessment and Research 2009; Couturier et al. 2020; Danish Health Authority 2016a, 2016b; Haute Autorité de Santé 2010; Golden et al. 2015a; Hackert et al. 2020; Hay et al. 2014; Herpertz et al. 2020; Hilbert et al. 2017; Hornberger et al. 2021; Lock et al. 2015a; National Guideline Alliance (UK) 2020; Ozier et al. 2011; Resmark et al. 2019; Royal Colleges of Psychiatrists 2014).

Rating the Strength of Supporting Research Evidence

Strength of supporting research evidence describes the level of confidence that findings from scientific observation and testing of an effect of an intervention reflect the true effect. Confidence is enhanced by such factors as rigorous study design and minimal potential for study bias.

Ratings were determined, in accordance with the Agency for Healthcare Research and Quality (AHRQ)'s Methods Guide for Effectiveness and Comparative Effectiveness Reviews (Agency for Healthcare Research and Quality 2014), by the methodologist (L.J.F.) and reviewed by members of the SRG and GWG. Available clinical trials were assessed across four primary domains: risk of bias, consistency of findings across studies, directness of the effect on a specific health outcome, and precision of the estimate of effect.

The ratings are defined as follows:

- High (denoted by the letter A)=High confidence that the evidence reflects the true effect. Further research is very unlikely to change our confidence in the estimate of effect.
- Moderate (denoted by the letter B)=Moderate confidence that the evidence reflects the true effect. Further research may change our confidence in the estimate of effect and may change the estimate.
- Low (denoted by the letter C)=Low confidence that the evidence reflects the true effect. Further research is likely to change our confidence in the estimate of effect and is likely to change the estimate.

The AHRQ has an additional category of *insufficient* for evidence that is unavailable or does not permit estimation of an effect. The APA uses the *low* rating when evidence is insufficient because there is low confidence in the conclusion and further research, if conducted, would likely change the estimated effect or confidence in the estimated effect.

Rating the Strength of Guideline Statements

Each guideline statement is separately rated to indicate strength of recommendation and strength of supporting research evidence. *Strength of recommendation* describes the level of confidence that potential benefits of an intervention outweigh potential harms. This level of confidence is informed by available evidence, which includes evidence from clinical trials as well as expert opinion and patient values and preferences. As described in the section "Rating the Strength of Supporting Research Evidence," this rating is a consensus judgment of the authors of the guideline and is endorsed by the APA Board of Trustees.

There are two possible ratings: recommendation or suggestion. A *recommendation* (denoted by the numeral 1 after the guideline statement) indicates confidence that the benefits of the intervention clearly outweigh harms. A *suggestion* (denoted by the numeral 2 after the guideline statement) indicates greater uncertainty. Although the benefits of the statement are still viewed as outweighing the harms, the balance of benefits and harms is more difficult to judge or either the benefits or the harms may be less clear. With a suggestion, patient values and preferences may be more variable, and this can influence the clinical decision that is ultimately made. These strengths of recommendation correspond to ratings of *strong* or *weak* (also termed *conditional)* as defined under the GRADE method for rating recommendations in clinical practice guidelines (described in publications such as Guyatt et al. 2008 and others available on the Web site of the GRADE Working Group at www.gradeworkinggroup.org).

When a negative statement is made, ratings of strength of recommendation should be understood as meaning the inverse of the above (e.g., *recommendation* indicates confidence that harms clearly outweigh benefits).

The GWG determined ratings of strength of recommendation by a modified Delphi method using blind iterative voting and discussion. In order for the GWG members to be able to ask for clarifications about the evidence, the wording of statements, or the process, the vice-chair of the GWG served as a resource and did not vote on statements. The chair and other formally appointed GWG members were eligible to vote.

In weighing potential benefits and harms, GWG members considered the strength of supporting research evidence, their own clinical experiences and opinions, and patient preferences. For recommendations, at least 13 out of 14 members must have voted to recommend the intervention or assessment after four rounds of voting, and at most 1 member was allowed to vote other than "recommend" the intervention or assessment. On the basis of the discussion among the GWG members, adjustments to the wording of recommendations could be made between the voting rounds. If this level of consensus was not achieved, the GWG could have agreed to make a suggestion rather than a recommendation. No suggestion or statement could have been made if 3 or more members voted "no statement." Differences of opinion within the GWG about ratings of strength of recommendation, if any, are described in the subsection of Appendix G, "Balancing of Potential Benefits and Harms in Rating the Strength of the Guideline Statements and Quality Measurement Considerations," for each statement.

External Review

This guideline was made available for review from October 5, 2021, to November 12, 2021, by stakeholders, including the APA membership, scientific and clinical experts, allied organizations, and the public. In addition, a number of patient advocacy organizations were invited for input. 108 individuals and 26 organizations submitted comments on the guideline (see the section "Individuals and Organizations That Submitted Comments" for a list of those who wished to be acknowledged in the guideline). The Chair and Co-chair of the GWG reviewed and addressed all comments received; substantive issues were reviewed by the GWG.

Funding and Approval

This guideline development project was funded and supported by the APA without any involvement of industry or external funding. The guideline was submitted to the APA Assembly and APA Board of Trustees and approved on March 21, 2022 and April 6, 2022, respectively.

References

References
Academy for Eating Disorders Medical Care Standards Committee: Eating Disorders: A Guide to Medical Care. AED Report, 4th Edition. Reston, VA, Academy for Eating Disorders, 2021

Academy for Eating Disorders Nutrition Working Group: Guidebook for Nutrition Treatment of Eating Disorders. Reston, VA, Academy for Eating Disorders, 2021

Accurso EC, Waller G: A brief session-by-session measure of eating disorder psychopathology for children and adolescents: development and psychometric properties of the Eating Disorder-15 for Youth (ED-15-Y). Int J Eat Disord 54(4):569–577, 2021a 33331681

Accurso EC, Waller G: Concordance between youth and caregiver report of eating disorder psychopathology: development and psychometric properties of the Eating Disorder-15 for Parents/Caregivers (ED-15-P). Int J Eat Disord 54(7):1302–1306, 2021b 34021612

Acevedo A, Garnick DW, Dunigan R, et al: Performance measures and racial/ethnic disparities in the treatment of substance use disorders. J Stud Alcohol Drugs 76(1):57–67, 2015 25486394

Achamrah N, Coëffier M, Rimbert A, et al: Micronutrient status in 153 patients with anorexia nervosa. Nutrients 9(3):225, 2017 28257095

Afifi TO, Sareen J, Fortier J, et al: Child maltreatment and eating disorders among men and women in adulthood: results from a nationally representative United States sample. Int J Eat Disord 50(11):1281–1296, 2017 28990206

Agency for Healthcare Research and Quality: Methods Guide for Effectiveness and Comparative Effectiveness Reviews (AHRQ Publ No 10~14~-EHC063-EF). Rockville, MD, Agency for Healthcare Research and Quality, 2014

Agostino H, Erdstein J, Di Meglio G: Shifting paradigms: continuous nasogastric feeding with high caloric intakes in anorexia nervosa. J Adolesc Health 53(5):590–594, 2013 23871800

Agostino H, Burstein B, Moubayed D, et al: Trends in the incidence of new-onset anorexia nervosa and atypical anorexia nervosa among youth during the COVID-19 pandemic in Canada. JAMA Netw Open 4(12):e2137395, 2021 34874405

Agras WS, Bohon C: Cognitive behavioral therapy for the eating disorders. Annu Rev Clin Psychol 17:417–438, 2021 33962536

Agras WS, Dorian B, Kirkley BG: Imipramine in the treatment of bulimia: a double-blind controlled study. Int J Eat Disord 6(1):29–38, 1987

Agras WS, Schneider JA, Arnow B, et al: Cognitive-behavioral and response-prevention treatments for bulimia nervosa. J Consult Clin Psychol 57(2):215–221, 1989 2708607

Agras WS, Rossiter EM, Arnow B, et al: Pharmacologic and cognitive-behavioral treatment for bulimia nervosa: a controlled comparison. Am J Psychiatry 149(1):82–87, 1992 1728190

Agras WS, Rossiter EM, Arnow B, et al: One-year follow-up of psychosocial and pharmacologic treatments for bulimia nervosa. J Clin Psychiatry 55(5):179–183, 1994a 8071266

Agras WS, Telch CF, Arnow B, et al: Weight loss, cognitive-behavioral, and desipramine treatments in binge eating disorder: an additive design. Behav Ther 25(2):225–238, 1994b

Agras WS, Telch CF, Arnow B, et al: Does interpersonal therapy help patients with binge eating disorder who fail to respond to cognitive-behavioral therapy? J Consult Clin Psychol 63(3):356–360, 1995 7608347

Agras WS, Walsh T, Fairburn CG, et al: A multicenter comparison of cognitive-behavioral therapy and interpersonal psychotherapy for bulimia nervosa. Arch Gen Psychiatry 57(5):459–466, 2000 10807486

Agras WS, Lock J, Brandt H, et al: Comparison of 2 family therapies for adolescent anorexia nervosa: a randomized parallel trial. JAMA Psychiatry 71(11):1279–1286, 2014 25250660

Ahn J, Lee JH, Jung YC: Predictors of suicide attempts in individuals with eating disorders. Suicide Life Threat Behav 49(3):789–797, 2019 29882994

Alegria M, Woo M, Cao Z, et al: Prevalence and correlates of eating disorders in Latinos in the United States. Int J Eat Disord 40(Suppl):S15–S21, 2007 17584870

Alfonsson S, Parling T, Ghaderi A: Group behavioral activation for patients with severe obesity and binge eating disorder: a randomized controlled trial. Behav Modif 39(2):270–294, 2015 25268019

Ali K, Farrer L, Fassnacht DB, et al: Perceived barriers and facilitators towards help-seeking for eating disorders: a systematic review. Int J Eat Disord 50(1):9–21, 2017 27526643

Allan E, Le Grange D, Sawyer SM, et al: Parental expressed emotion during two forms of family based treatment for adolescent anorexia nervosa. Eur Eat Disord Rev 26(1):46–52, 2018 29105211

Allen HN, Craighead LW: Appetite monitoring in the treatment of binge eating disorder. Behav Ther 30(2):253–272, 1999

Allen DB, Merchant N, Miller BS, Backeljauw PF: Evolution and future of growth plate therapeutics. Horm Res Paediatr 94(9–10):319–332, 2021 34758467

American College of Obstetricians and Gynecologists: ACOG committee opinion No. 740: gynecologic care for adolescents and young women with eating disorders. Obstet Gynecol 131(6):e205–e213, 2018 29794682

American Geriatrics Society Expert Panel on Person-Centered Care: Person-centered care: a definition and essential elements. J Am Geriatr Soc 64(1):15–18, 2016 26626262

American Psychiatric Association: Diagnostic and Statistical Manual of Mental Disorders, 4th Edition. Arlington, VA, American Psychiatric Association, 1994

American Psychiatric Association: American Psychiatric Association Practice Guideline for the Treatment of Patients With Eating Disorders, 3rd Edition. Washington, DC, American Psychiatric Publishing, 2006

American Psychiatric Association: Diagnostic and Statistical Manual of Mental Disorders, 5th Edition. Arlington, VA, American Psychiatric Association, 2013

American Psychiatric Association: American Psychiatric Association Practice Guidelines for the Psychiatric Evaluation of Adults, 3rd Edition. Arlington, VA, American Psychiatric Association Publishing, 2016

American Psychiatric Association: Diagnostic and Statistical Manual of Mental Disorders, 5th Edition, Text Revision. Washington, DC, American Psychiatric Association, 2022

Anand P, Mehler PS: Osteoporosis recovery in severe anorexia nervosa: a case report. J Eat Disord 7:38, 2019 31719982

Anastasiadou D, Folkvord F, Lupiañez-Villanueva F: A systematic review of mHealth interventions for the support of eating disorders. Eur Eat Disord Rev 26(5):394–416, 2018 29927004

Andersen L, LaRosa C, Gih DE: Reexamining the role of electroconvulsive therapy in anorexia nervosa in adolescents. J ECT 33(4):294–296, 2017 28471772

Anderson KE, Byrne CE, Crosby RD, et al: Utilizing telehealth to deliver family based treatment for adolescent anorexia nervosa. Int J Eat Disord 50(10):1235–1238, 2017 28801943

Andrews JC, Schünemann HJ, Oxman AD, et al: GRADE guidelines: 15. Going from evidence to recommendation-determinants of a recommendation's direction and strength. J Clin Epidemiol 66(7):726–735, 2013 23570745

Arbel R, Latzer Y, Koren D: Revisiting poor insight into illness in anorexia nervosa: true unawareness or conscious disagreement? J Psychiatr Pract 20(2):85–93, 2014 24638043

Arcelus J, Mitchell AJ, Wales J, et al: Mortality rates in patients with anorexia nervosa and other eating disorders: a meta-analysis of 36 studies. Arch Gen Psychiatry 68(7):724–731, 2011 21727255

Asch DA, Buresh J, Allison KC, et al: Trends in US patients receiving care for eating disorders and other common behavioral health conditions before and during the COVID-19 pandemic. JAMA Netw Open 4(11):e2134913, 2021 34783829

Atti AR, Mastellari T, Valente S, et al: Compulsory treatments in eating disorders: a systematic review and meta-analysis. Eat Weight Disord 26(4):1037–1048, 2021 33099675

Attia E, Walsh BT: Behavioral management for anorexia nervosa. N Engl J Med 360(5):500–506, 2009 19179317

Attia E, Kaplan AS, Walsh BT, et al: Olanzapine versus placebo for out-patients with anorexia nervosa. Psychol Med 41(10):2177–2182, 2011 21426603 Erratum in: Am J Psychiatry 176(6):489, 2019

Attia E, Steinglass JE, Walsh BT, et al: Olanzapine versus placebo in adult outpatients with anorexia nervosa: a randomized clinical trial. Am J Psychiatry 176(6):449–456, 2019 30654643

Auger N, Potter BJ, Ukah UV, et al: Anorexia nervosa and the long-term risk of mortality in women. World Psychiatry 20(3):448–449, 2021 34505367

Avila JT, Golden NH, Aye T: Eating disorder screening in transgender youth. J Adolesc Health 65(6):815–817, 2019 31500946

Bachar E, Latzer Y, Kreitler S, et al: Empirical comparison of two psychological therapies: self psychology and cognitive orientation in the treatment of anorexia and bulimia. J Psychother Pract Res 8(2):115–128, 1999 10079459

Bahji A, Mazhar MN, Hudson CC, et al: Prevalence of substance use disorder comorbidity among individuals with eating disorders: a systematic review and meta-analysis. Psychiatry Res 273:58–66, 2019 30640052

Bailer U, de Zwaan M, Leisch F, et al: Guided self-help versus cognitive-behavioral group therapy in the treatment of bulimia nervosa. Int J Eat Disord 35(4):522–537, 2004 15101068

Ball J, Mitchell P: A randomized controlled study of cognitive behavior therapy and behavioral family therapy for anorexia nervosa patients. Eat Disord 12(4):303–314, 2004 16864523

Balshem H, Helfand M, Schünemann HJ, et al: GRADE guidelines: 3. Rating the quality of evidence. J Clin Epidemiol 64(4):401–406, 2011 21208779

Banasiak SJ, Paxton SJ, Hay P: Guided self-help for bulimia nervosa in primary care: a randomized controlled trial. Psychol Med 35(9):1283–1294, 2005 16168151

Bang L, Tamnes CK, Norbom LB, et al: Associations of age, body mass index and biochemical parameters with brain morphology in patients with anorexia nervosa. Eur Eat Disord Rev 29(1):74–85, 2021 33125776

Barakat S, Maguire S, Smith KE, et al: Evaluating the role of digital intervention design in treatment outcomes and adherence to eTherapy programs for eating disorders: a systematic review and meta-analysis. Int J Eat Disord 52(10):1077–1094, 2019 31328815

Barbarich NC, McConaha CW, Halmi KA, et al: Use of nutritional supplements to increase the efficacy of fluoxetine in the treatment of anorexia nervosa. Int J Eat Disord 35(1):10–15, 2004 14705152

Baudinet J, Eisler I, Dawson L, et al: Multi-family therapy for eating disorders: a systematic scoping review of the quantitative and qualitative findings. Int J Eat Disord 54(12):2095–2120, 2021 34672007

Bauer S, Okon E, Meermann R, et al: Technology-enhanced maintenance of treatment gains in eating disorders: efficacy of an intervention delivered via text messaging. J Consult Clin Psychol 80(4):700–706, 2012 22545736

Ben-Porath D, Duthu F, Luo T, et al: Dialectical behavioral therapy: an update and review of the existing treatment models adapted for adults with eating disorders. Eat Disord 28(2):101–121, 2020 32129724

Berends T, Boonstra N, van Elburg A: Relapse in anorexia nervosa: a systematic review and meta-analysis. Curr Opin Psychiatry 31(6):445–455, 2018 30113325

Beumont PJ, Russell JD, Touyz SW, et al: Intensive nutritional counselling in bulimia nervosa: a role for supplementation with fluoxetine? Aust N Z J Psychiatry 31(4):514–524, 1997 9272261

Biney H, Astbury S, Haines A, et al: A novel 'practical body image' therapy for adolescent inpatients with anorexia nervosa: a randomised controlled trial. Eat Weight Disord 26(6):1825–1834, 2021 32949382

Biney H, Giles E, Hutt M, et al: Self-esteem as a catalyst for change in adolescent inpatients with anorexia nervosa: a pilot randomised controlled trial. Eat Weight Disord 27(1):189–198, 2022 33713335

Bissada H, Tasca GA, Barber AM, et al: Olanzapine in the treatment of low body weight and obsessive thinking in women with anorexia nervosa: a randomized, double-blind, placebo-controlled trial. Am J Psychiatry 165(10):1281–1288, 2008 18558642

Blalock DV, Le Grange D, Johnson C, et al: Pilot assessment of a virtual intensive outpatient program for adults with eating disorders. Eur Eat Disord Rev 28(6):789–795, 2020 32844501

Blissett J, Haycraft E: Parental eating disorder symptoms and observations of mealtime interactions with children. J Psychosom Res 70(4):368–371, 2011 21414457

Bloch M, Ish-Shalom S, Greenman Y, et al: Dehydroepiandrosterone treatment effects on weight, bone density, bone metabolism and mood in women suffering from anorexia nervosa-a pilot study. Psychiatry Res 200(2–3):544–549, 2012 22858403

Bohn K, Doll HA, Cooper Z, et al: The measurement of impairment due to eating disorder psychopathology. Behav Res Ther 46(10):1105–1110, 2008 18710699

Botella J, Sepúlveda AR, Huang H, et al: A meta-analysis of the diagnostic accuracy of the SCOFF. Span J Psychol 16:E92, 2013 24230955

Brambilla F, Garcia CS, Fassino S, et al: Olanzapine therapy in anorexia nervosa: psychobiological effects. Int Clin Psychopharmacol 22(4):197–204, 2007 17519642

Brambilla F, Samek L, Company M, et al: Multivariate therapeutic approach to binge-eating disorder: combined nutritional, psychological and pharmacological treatment. Int Clin Psychopharmacol 24(6):312–317, 2009 19794312

Braude MR, Con D, Clayton-Chubb D, et al: Acute medical stabilisation of adults with anorexia nervosa: experience of a defined interdisciplinary model of care. Intern Med J 50(1):77–85, 2020 31059162

Brelet L, Flaudias V, Désert M, et al: Stigmatization toward people with anorexia nervosa, bulimia nervosa, and binge eating disorder: a scoping review. Nutrients 13(8):2834, 2021 34444994

Brennan MA, Whelton WJ, Sharpe D: Benefits of yoga in the treatment of eating disorders: results of a randomized controlled trial. Eat Disord 28(4):438–457, 2020 32182190

Brewerton TD: The use and scoring of the Kids' Eating Disorders Survey (KEDS). Eat Disord 9(1):71–74, 2001 16864375

Brewerton TD, D'Agostino M: Adjunctive use of olanzapine in the treatment of avoidant restrictive food intake disorder in children and adolescents in an eating disorders program. J Child Adolesc Psychopharmacol 27(10):920–922, 2017 29068721

Brewerton TD, Duncan AE: Associations between attention deficit hyperactivity disorder and eating disorders by gender: results from the national comorbidity survey replication. Eur Eat Disord Rev 24(6):536–540, 2016 27480884

Bristow C, Meurer C, Simmonds J, et al: Anti-obesity public health messages and risk factors for disordered eating: a systematic review. Health Promot Int 35(6):1551–1569, 2020 32150266

Brito JP, Domecq JP, Murad MH, et al: The Endocrine Society guidelines: when the confidence cart goes before the evidence horse. J Clin Endocrinol Metab 98(8):3246–3252, 2013 23783104

Brown RF, Bartrop R, Birmingham CL: Immunological disturbance and infectious disease in anorexia nervosa: a review. Acta Neuropsychiatr 20(3):117–128, 2008 26951035

Brownley KA, Von Holle A, Hamer RM, et al: A double-blind, randomized pilot trial of chromium picolinate for binge eating disorder: results of the Binge Eating and Chromium (BEACh) study. J Psychosom Res 75(1):36–42, 2013 23751236

Bryant-Waugh R, Micali N, Cooke L, et al: Development of the Pica, ARFID, and Rumination Disorder Interview, a multi-informant, semi-structured interview of feeding disorders across the lifespan: a pilot study for ages 10–22. Int J Eat Disord 52(4):378–387, 2019 30312485

Byford S, Barrett B, Roberts C, et al: Economic evaluation of a randomised controlled trial for anorexia nervosa in adolescents. Br J Psychiatry 191:436–440, 2007 17978324

Byrne S, Wade T, Hay P, et al: A randomised controlled trial of three psychological treatments for anorexia nervosa. Psychol Med 47(16):2823–2833, 2017 28552083

Cachelin FM, Striegel-Moore RH: Help seeking and barriers to treatment in a community sample of Mexican American and European American women with eating disorders. Int J Eat Disord 39(2):154–161, 2006 16252278

Cachelin FM, Gil-Rivas V, Palmer B, et al: Randomized controlled trial of a culturally adapted program for Latinas with binge eating. Psychol Serv 16(3):504–512, 2019 29620392

Carrard I, Crépin C, Rouget P, et al: Randomised controlled trial of a guided self-help treatment on the internet for binge eating disorder. Behav Res Ther 49(8):482–491, 2011 21641580

Carter FA, Jordan J, McIntosh VV, et al: The long-term efficacy of three psychotherapies for anorexia nervosa: a randomized, controlled trial. Int J Eat Disord 44(7):647–654, 2011 21997429

Carter JC, Fairburn CG: Cognitive-behavioral self-help for binge eating disorder: a controlled effectiveness study. J Consult Clin Psychol 66(4):616–623, 1998 9735577

Carter JC, Olmsted MP, Kaplan AS, et al: Self-help for bulimia nervosa: a randomized controlled trial. Am J Psychiatry 160(5):973–978, 2003 12727703

Carter JC, McFarlane TL, Bewell C, et al: Maintenance treatment for anorexia nervosa: a comparison of cognitive behavior therapy and treatment as usual. Int J Eat Disord 42(3):202–207, 2009 18949764

Carter JC, Kenny TE, Singleton C, et al: Dialectical behavior therapy self-help for binge-eating disorder: a randomized controlled study. Int J Eat Disord 53(3):451–460, 2020 31821592

Cass K, McGuire C, Bjork I, et al: Medical complications of anorexia nervosa. Psychosomatics 61(6):625–631, 2020 32778424

Castelnuovo G, Manzoni GM, Villa V, et al: Brief strategic therapy vs cognitive behavioral therapy for the inpatient and telephone-based outpatient treatment of binge eating disorder: the STRATOB randomized controlled clinical trial. Clin Pract Epidemiol Ment Health 7:29–37, 2011 21559234

Catalan Agency for Health Technology Assessment and Research: Clinical Practice Guideline for Eating Disorders (Clinical Practice Guideline in the NHS: CAHTA; No.2006/05-01). Madrid, Quality Plan for the National Health System of the Ministry of Health and Consumer Affairs, Catalan Agency for Health Technology Assessment and Research, 2009

Center for Health Policy/Center for Primary Care and Outcomes Research and Battelle Memorial Institute: Quality Indicator Measure Development, Implementation, Maintenance, and Retirement. Contract No 290–04–0020. Rockville, MD, Agency for Healthcare Research and Quality, 2011

Chao AM, Wadden TA, Faulconbridge LF, et al: Binge-eating disorder and the outcome of bariatric surgery in a prospective, observational study: two-year results. Obesity (Silver Spring) 24(11):2327–2333, 2016 27616677

Chen E, Touyz SW, Beumont PJ, et al: Comparison of group and individual cognitive-behavioral therapy for patients with bulimia nervosa. Int J Eat Disord 33(3):241–254, discussion 255–256, 2003 12655619

Chen EY, Weissman JA, Zeffiro TA, et al: Family based therapy for young adults with anorexia nervosa restores weight. Int J Eat Disord 49(7):701–707, 2016 27037965

Childress AC, Brewerton TD, Hodges EL, et al: The Kids' Eating Disorders Survey (KEDS): a study of middle school students. J Am Acad Child Adolesc Psychiatry 32(4):843–850, 1993 8340308

Chung A, Vieira D, Donley T, et al: Adolescent peer influence on eating behaviors via social media: scoping review. J Med Internet Res 23(6):e19697, 2021 34081018

Ciao AC, Accurso EC, Fitzsimmons-Craft EE, et al: Family functioning in two treatments for adolescent anorexia nervosa. Int J Eat Disord 48(1):81–90, 2015 24902822

Cierpka M, Grande T, Rudolf G, et al: The operationalized psychodynamic diagnostics system: clinical relevance, reliability and validity. Psychopathology 40(4):209–220, 2007 17396047

Cipriani A, Zhou X, Del Giovane C, et al: Comparative efficacy and tolerability of antidepressants for major depressive disorder in children and adolescents: a network meta-analysis. Lancet 388(10047):881–890, 2016 27289172

Claudino AM, de Oliveira IR, Appolinario JC, et al: Double-blind, randomized, placebo-controlled trial of topiramate plus cognitive-behavior therapy in binge-eating disorder. J Clin Psychiatry 68(9):1324–1332, 2007 17915969

Cleary BS, Gaudiani JL, Mehler PS: Interpreting the complete blood count in anorexia nervosa. Eat Disord 18(2):132–139, 2010 20390616

Cliffe C, Shetty H, Himmerich H, et al: Suicide attempts requiring hospitalization in patients with eating disorders: a retrospective cohort study. Int J Eat Disord 53(5):458–465, 2020 32043625

Coelho JS, Suen J, Clark BA, et al: Eating disorder diagnoses and symptom presentation in transgender youth: a scoping review. Curr Psychiatry Rep 21(11):107, 2019 31617014

Coffino JA, Udo T, Grilo CM: Rates of help-seeking in US adults with lifetime DSM-5 eating disorders: prevalence across diagnoses and differences by sex and ethnicity/race. Mayo Clin Proc 94(8):1415–1426, 2019 31324401

Coffino JA, Grilo CM, Udo T: Childhood food neglect and adverse experiences associated with DSM-5 eating disorders in U.S. national sample. J Psychiatr Res 127:75–79, 2020 32502721

Compare A, Calugi S, Marchesini G, et al: Emotionally focused group therapy and dietary counseling in binge eating disorder: effect on eating disorder psychopathology and quality of life. Appetite 71:361–368, 2013a 24060270

Compare A, Calugi S, Marchesini G, et al: Emotion-focused therapy and dietary counseling for obese patients with binge eating disorder: a propensity score-adjusted study. Psychother Psychosom 82(3):193–194, 2013b 23549048

Cooper M, Guarda AS, Petterway F, et al: Change in normative eating self-efficacy is associated with six-month weight restoration following inpatient treatment for anorexia nervosa. Eat Behav 42:101518, 2021 33989938

Cooper PJ, Steere J: A comparison of two psychological treatments for bulimia nervosa: implications for models of maintenance. Behav Res Ther 33(8):875–885, 1995 7487847

Cooper Z, Fairburn CG: The evolution of "enhanced" cognitive behavior therapy for eating disorders: learning from treatment nonresponse. Cognit Behav Pract 18(3):394–402, 2011 23814455

Cope S, Zhang J, Saletan S, et al: A process for assessing the feasibility of a network meta-analysis: a case study of everolimus in combination with hormonal therapy versus chemotherapy for advanced breast cancer. BMC Med 12:93, 2014 24898705

Cotton MA, Ball C, Robinson P: Four simple questions can help screen for eating disorders. J Gen Intern Med 18(1):53–56, 2003 12534764

Council of Medical Specialty Societies: Principles for the Development of Specialty Society Clinical Guidelines. Chicago, IL, Council of Medical Specialty Societies, 2012

Court A, Mulder C, Kerr M, et al: Investigating the effectiveness, safety and tolerability of quetiapine in the treatment of anorexia nervosa in young people: a pilot study. J Psychiatr Res 44(15):1027–1034, 2010 20447652

Couturier J, Isserlin L, Norris M, et al: Canadian practice guidelines for the treatment of children and adolescents with eating disorders. J Eat Disord 8:4, 2020 32021688

Crisp AH, Norton K, Gowers S, et al: A controlled study of the effect of therapies aimed at adolescent and family psychopathology in anorexia nervosa. Br J Psychiatry 159:325–333, 1991 1958942

Crosby RD, Mitchell JE, Raymond N, et al: Survival analysis of response to group psychotherapy in bulimia nervosa. Int J Eat Disord 13(4):359–368, 1993 8490638

Cucchi A, Ryan D, Konstantakopoulos G, et al: Lifetime prevalence of non-suicidal self-injury in patients with eating disorders: a systematic review and meta-analysis. Psychol Med 46(7):1345–1358, 2016 26954514

da Silva JSV, Seres DS, Sabino K, et al: ASPEN consensus recommendations for refeeding syndrome. Nutr Clin Pract 35(2):178–195, 2020 32115791 Erratum in: Nutr Clin Pract 35(3):584–585, 2020 32383800

Dahlenburg SC, Gleaves DH, Hutchinson AD: Anorexia nervosa and perfectionism: a meta-analysis. Int J Eat Disord 52(3):219–229, 2019 30632629

Dalle Grave R, Calugi S: Cognitive Behavior Therapy for Adolescents With Eating Disorders. New York, Guilford, 2020

Dalle Grave R, Calugi S, Conti M, et al: Inpatient cognitive behaviour therapy for anorexia nervosa: a randomized controlled trial. Psychother Psychosom 82(6):390–398, 2013a 24060628

Dalle Grave R, Calugi S, Doll HA, et al: Enhanced cognitive behaviour therapy for adolescents with anorexia nervosa: an alternative to family therapy? Behav Res Ther 51(1):R9–R12, 2013b 23123081

Dalle Grave R, Conti M, Sartirana M, et al: Enhanced cognitive behaviour therapy for adolescents with eating disorders: a systematic review of current status and future perspectives. Ijedo 3:1–11, 2021

Daniel SIF, Poulsen S, Lunn S: Client attachment in a randomized clinical trial of psychoanalytic and cognitive-behavioral psychotherapy for bulimia nervosa: outcome moderation and change. Psychotherapy (Chic) 53(2):174–184, 2016 26950692

Danish Health Authority: National Clinical Guideline for the Treatment of Anorexia Nervosa. København, Denmark, Danish Health Authority, October 2016a

Danish Health Authority: National Clinical Guideline for the Treatment of Moderate and Severe Bulimia. København, Denmark, Danish Health Authority, March 2016b

Dare C, Eisler I, Russell G, et al: The clinical and theoretical impact of a controlled trial of family therapy in anorexia nervosa. J Marital Fam Ther 16(1):39–57, 1990

Dare C, Eisler I, Russell G, et al: Psychological therapies for adults with anorexia nervosa: randomised controlled trial of out-patient treatments. Br J Psychiatry 178:216–221, 2001 11230031

Dastan B, Afshar Zanjani S, Froueddin Adl A, et al: The effectiveness of dialectical behaviour therapy for treating women with obesity suffering from BED: a feasibility and pilot study. Clin Psychol 24:133–142, 2020

Davis R, McVey G, Heinmaa M, et al: Sequencing of cognitive-behavioral treatments for bulimia nervosa. Int J Eat Disord 25(4):361–374, 1999 10202647

Day AS, Yao CK, Costello SP, et al: Food-related quality of life in adults with inflammatory bowel disease is associated with restrictive eating behaviour, disease activity and surgery: a prospective multicentre observational study. J Hum Nutr Diet 35(1):234–244, 2022 34008222

Day S, Bussey K, Trompeter N, et al: The impact of teasing and bullying victimization on disordered eating and body image disturbance among adolescents: a systematic review. Trauma Violence Abuse 23(3):985–1006, 2022 33461439

De Souza MJ, Nattiv A, Joy E, et al: 2014 Female Athlete Triad coalition consensus statement on treatment and return to play of the female athlete triad: 1st international conference held in San Francisco, California, May 2012 and 2nd international conference held in Indianapolis, Indiana, May 2013. Br J Sports Med 48(4):289, 2014 24463911

de Zwaan M, Mitchell JE, Crosby RD, et al: Short-term cognitive behavioral treatment does not improve outcome of a comprehensive very-low-calorie diet program in obese women with binge eating disorder. Behav Ther 36(1):89–99, 2005

de Zwaan M, Herpertz S, Zipfel S, et al: Effect of internet-based guided self-help vs individual face-to-face treatment on full or subsyndromal binge eating disorder in overweight or obese patients: the INTERBED randomized clinical trial. JAMA Psychiatry 74(10):987–995, 2017 28768334

del Valle MF, Pérez M, Santana-Sosa E, et al: Does resistance training improve the functional capacity and well being of very young anorexic patients? A randomized controlled trial. J Adolesc Health 46(4):352–358, 2010 20307824

Dempfle A, Herpertz-Dahlmann B, Timmesfeld N, et al: Predictors of the resumption of menses in adolescent anorexia nervosa. BMC Psychiatry 13:308, 2013 24238469

Devlin MJ, Goldfein JA, Petkova E, et al: Cognitive behavioral therapy and fluoxetine as adjuncts to group behavioral therapy for binge eating disorder. Obes Res 13(6):1077–1088, 2005 15976151

Devlin MJ, Goldfein JA, Petkova E, et al: Cognitive behavioral therapy and fluoxetine for binge eating disorder: two-year follow-up. Obesity (Silver Spring) 15(7):1702–1709, 2007 17636088

Dimitropoulos G, Landers AL, Freeman V, et al: Open trial of family based treatment of anorexia nervosa for transition age youth. J Can Acad Child Adolesc Psychiatry 27(1):50–61, 2018 29375633

Dittmer N, Jacobi C, Voderholzer U: Compulsive exercise in eating disorders: proposal for a definition and a clinical assessment. J Eat Disord 6:42, 2018 30505444

Divasta AD, Feldman HA, Giancaterino C, et al: The effect of gonadal and adrenal steroid therapy on skeletal health in adolescents and young women with anorexia nervosa. Metabolism 61(7):1010–1020, 2012 22257645

DiVasta AD, Feldman HA, Beck TJ, et al: Does hormone replacement normalize bone geometry in adolescents with anorexia nervosa? J Bone Miner Res 29(1):151–157, 2014 23744513

Djulbegovic B, Trikalinos TA, Roback J, et al: Impact of quality of evidence on the strength of recommendations: an empirical study. BMC Health Serv Res 9:120, 2009 19622148

Dobinson A, Cooper M, Quesnel D: Safe Exercise at Every Stage (SEES) guideline—a clinical tool for treating and managing dysfunctional exercise in eating disorders. Safe Exercise at Every Stage, 2019. Available at: https://www.safeexerciseateverystage.com/access-sees-guidelines. Accessed January 17, 2022.

Dobrescu SR, Dinkler L, Gillberg C, et al: Anorexia nervosa: 30-year outcome. Br J Psychiatry 216(2):97–104, 2020 31113504

Drake R, Skinner J, Goldman HH: What explains the diffusion of treatments for mental illness? Am J Psychiatry 165(11):1385–1392, 2008 18981070

Duffy ME, Calzo JP, Lopez E, et al: Measurement and construct validity of the Eating Disorder Examination Questionnaire Short Form in a transgender and gender diverse community sample. Psychol Assess 33(5):459–463, 2021 33646808

Dufresne L, Bussières E-L, Bédard A, et al: Personality traits in adolescents with eating disorder: a meta-analytic review. Int J Eat Disord 53(2):157–173, 2020 31633223

Dumont E, Jansen A, Kroes D, et al: A new cognitive behavior therapy for adolescents with avoidant/restrictive food intake disorder in a day treatment setting: a clinical case series. Int J Eat Disord 52(4):447–458, 2019 30805969

Duncan AE, Ziobrowski HN, Nicol G: The prevalence of past 12-month and lifetime DSM-IV eating disorders by BMI category in US men and women. Eur Eat Disord Rev 25(3):165–171, 2017 28127825

Durand MA, King M: Specialist treatment versus self-help for bulimia nervosa: a randomised controlled trial in general practice. Br J Gen Pract 53(490):371–377, 2003 12830564

Edakubo S, Fushimi K: Mortality and risk assessment for anorexia nervosa in acute-care hospitals: a nationwide administrative database analysis. BMC Psychiatry 20(1):19, 2020 31931765

Eddy KT, Tabri N, Thomas JJ, et al: Recovery from anorexia nervosa and bulimia nervosa at 22-year follow-up. J Clin Psychiatry 78(2):184–189, 2017 28002660

Eddy KT, Harshman SG, Becker KR, et al: Radcliffe ARFID workgroup: toward operationalization of research diagnostic criteria and directions for the field. Int J Eat Disord 52(4):361–366, 2019 30758864

Eichstadt M, Luzier J, Cho D, Weisenmuller C: Eating disorders in male athletes. Sports Health 12(4):327–333, 2020 32525767

Eielsen HP, Vrabel K, Hoffart A, et al: The 17-year outcome of 62 adult patients with longstanding eating disorders: a prospective study. Int J Eat Disord 54(5):841–850, 2021 33660895

Eisler I, Dare C, Russell GF, et al: Family and individual therapy in anorexia nervosa: a 5-year follow-up. Arch Gen Psychiatry 54(11):1025–1030, 1997 9366659

Eisler I, Dare C, Hodes M, et al: Family therapy for adolescent anorexia nervosa: the results of a controlled comparison of two family interventions. J Child Psychol Psychiatry 41(6):727–736, 2000 11039685

Eisler I, Simic M, Russell GF, et al: A randomised controlled treatment trial of two forms of family therapy in adolescent anorexia nervosa: a five-year follow-up. J Child Psychol Psychiatry 48(6):552–560, 2007 17537071

Eisler I, Simic M, Hodsoll J, et al: A pragmatic randomised multi-centre trial of multifamily and single family therapy for adolescent anorexia nervosa. BMC Psychiatry 16(1):422, 2016 27881106

El Ghoch M, Gatti D, Calugi S, et al: The association between weight gain/restoration and bone mineral density in adolescents with anorexia nervosa: a systematic review. Nutrients 8(12):769, 2016 27916839

Eldredge KL, Stewart Agras W, Arnow B, et al: The effects of extending cognitive-behavioral therapy for binge eating disorder among initial treatment nonresponders. Int J Eat Disord 21(4):347–352, 1997 9138046

Emery RL, Yoon C, Mason SM, et al: Childhood maltreatment and disordered eating attitudes and behaviors in adult men and women: findings from project EAT. Appetite 163:105224, 2021 33766616

Fairburn CG: Overcoming Binge Eating. New York, Guilford, 1995

Fairburn CG: Cognitive Behavior Therapy and Eating Disorders. New York, Guilford, 2008

Fairburn CG: Overcoming Binge Eating: The Proven Program to Learn Why You Binge and How You Can Stop, 2nd Edition. New York, Guilford, 2013

Fairburn CG, Jones R, Peveler RC, et al: Three psychological treatments for bulimia nervosa: a comparative trial. Arch Gen Psychiatry 48(5):463–469, 1991 2021299

Fairburn CG, Jones R, Peveler RC, et al: Psychotherapy and bulimia nervosa: longer-term effects of interpersonal psychotherapy, behavior therapy, and cognitive behavior therapy. Arch Gen Psychiatry 50(6):419–428, 1993 8498876

Fairburn CG, Cooper Z, Shafran R: Cognitive behaviour therapy for eating disorders: a "transdiagnostic" theory and treatment. Behav Res Ther 41(5):509–528, 2003 12711261

Faje AT, Fazeli PK, Katzman DK, et al: Sclerostin levels and bone turnover markers in adolescents with anorexia nervosa and healthy adolescent girls. Bone 51(3):474–479, 2012 22728230

Faje AT, Fazeli PK, Miller KK, et al: Fracture risk and areal bone mineral density in adolescent females with anorexia nervosa. Int J Eat Disord 47(5):458–466, 2014 24430890

Farag F, Sims A, Strudwick K, et al: Avoidant/restrictive food intake disorder and autism spectrum disorder: clinical implications for assessment and management. Dev Med Child Neurol 64(2):176–182, 2022 34405406

Fassino S, Leombruni P, Daga G, et al: Efficacy of citalopram in anorexia nervosa: a pilot study. Eur Neuropsychopharmacol 12(5):453–459, 2002 12208563

Faust JP, Goldschmidt AB, Anderson KE, et al: Resumption of menses in anorexia nervosa during a course of family based treatment. J Eat Disord 1:12, 2013 24926411

Favaro A, Caregaro L, Tenconi E, et al: Time trends in age at onset of anorexia nervosa and bulimia nervosa. J Clin Psychiatry 70(12):1715–1721, 2009 20141711

Fazeli PK, Lawson EA, Prabhakaran R, et al: Effects of recombinant human growth hormone in anorexia nervosa: a randomized, placebo-controlled study. J Clin Endocrinol Metab 95(11):4889–4897, 2010 20668047

Fazeli PK, Wang IS, Miller KK, et al: Teriparatide increases bone formation and bone mineral density in adult women with anorexia nervosa. J Clin Endocrinol Metab 99(4):1322–1329, 2014 24456286

Feillet F, Bocquet A, Briend A, et al: Nutritional risks of ARFID (avoidant restrictive food intake disorders) and related behavior. Arch Pediatr 26(7):437–441, 2019 31500920

Feltner C, Peat C, Reddy S, et al: Screening for Eating Disorders in Adolescents and Adults: An Evidence Review for the U.S. Preventive Services Task Force. Evidence Synthesis No. 212. AHRQ Publ No 21-05284-EF-1. Rockville, MD, Agency for Healthcare Research and Quality, 2021

Fernandes-Taylor S, Harris AH: Comparing alternative specifications of quality measures: access to pharmacotherapy for alcohol use disorders. J Subst Abuse Treat 42(1):102–107, 2012 21839604

Fernández-Aranda F, Núñez A, Martínez C, et al: Internet-based cognitive-behavioral therapy for bulimia nervosa: a controlled study. Cyberpsychol Behav 12(1):37–41, 2009 19006463

Fernandez-del-Valle M, Larumbe-Zabala E, Villaseñor-Montarroso A, et al: Resistance training enhances muscular performance in patients with anorexia nervosa: a randomized controlled trial. Int J Eat Disord 47(6):601–609, 2014 24810684

Ferrell EL, Russin SE, Flint DD: Prevalence estimates of comorbid eating disorders and posttraumatic stress disorder: a quantitative synthesis. J Aggress Maltreat Trauma 31(2):264–282, 2020

Fichter MM, Krüger R, Rief W, et al: Fluvoxamine in prevention of relapse in bulimia nervosa: effects on eating-specific psychopathology. J Clin Psychopharmacol 16(1):9–18, 1996 8834413

Fichter MM, Leibl C, Krüger R, et al: Effects of fluvoxamine on depression, anxiety, and other areas of general psychopathology in bulimia nervosa. Pharmacopsychiatry 30(3):85–92, 1997 9211569

Fichter MM, Quadflieg N, Nisslmüller K, et al: Does internet-based prevention reduce the risk of relapse for anorexia nervosa? Behav Res Ther 50(3):180–190, 2012 22317754

Fichter MM, Quadflieg N, Lindner S: Internet-based relapse prevention for anorexia nervosa: nine-month follow-up. J Eat Disord 1:23, 2013 24999404

Fichter MM, Naab S, Voderholzer U, et al: Mortality in males as compared to females treated for an eating disorder: a large prospective controlled study. Eat Weight Disord 26(5):1627–1637, 2021 32789622

Fink M, Simons M, Tomasino K, et al: When is patient behavior indicative of avoidant restrictive food intake disorder (ARFID) vs reasonable response to digestive disease? Clin Gastroenterol Hepatol 20(6):1241–1250, 2022

Fisher MM, Rosen DS, Ornstein RM, et al: Characteristics of avoidant/restrictive food intake disorder in children and adolescents: a "new disorder" in DSM-5. J Adolesc Health 55(1):49–52, 2014 24506978

Fitzpatrick KK, Moye A, Hoste R, et al: Adolescent focused psychotherapy for adolescents with anorexia nervosa. J Contemp Psychother 40:31–39, 2010

Flanagin A, Frey T, Christiansen SL, et al: Updated guidance on the reporting of race and ethnicity in medical and science journals. JAMA 326(7):621–627, 2021 34402850

Fluoxetine Bulimia Nervosa Collaborative Study Group: Fluoxetine in the treatment of bulimia nervosa: a multicenter, placebo-controlled, double-blind trial. Arch Gen Psychiatry 49(2):139–147, 1992 1550466

Folke S, Daniel SI, Poulsen S, et al: Client attachment security predicts alliance in a randomized controlled trial of two psychotherapies for bulimia nervosa. Psychother Res 26(4):459–471, 2016 25869827

Foran AM, O'Donnell AT, Muldoon OT: Stigma of eating disorders and recovery-related outcomes: a systematic review. Eur Eat Disord Rev 28(4):385–397, 2020 32219911

Forbush KT, Richardson JH, Bohrer BK: Clinicians' practices regarding blind versus open weighing among patients with eating disorders. Int J Eat Disord 48(7):905–911, 2015 25504058

Forrest LN, Grilo CM, Udo T: Suicide attempts among people with eating disorders and adverse childhood experiences: results from a nationally representative sample of adults. Int J Eat Disord 54(3):326–335, 2021 33372308

Fortney JC, Unützer J, Wrenn G, et al: A tipping point for measurement-based care. Psychiatr Serv 68(2):179–188, 2017 27582237

Franko DL, Tabri N, Keshaviah A, et al: Predictors of long-term recovery in anorexia nervosa and bulimia nervosa: data from a 22-year longitudinal study. J Psychiatr Res 96:183–188, 2018 29078155

Fredericson M, Kussman A, Misra M, et al: The male athlete triad-a consensus statement from the Female and Male Athlete Triad Coalition Part II: diagnosis, treatment, and return-to-play. Clin J Sport Med 31(4):349–366, 2021 34091538

Frederiksen TC, Christiansen MK, Østergaard PC, et al: The QTc interval and risk of cardiac events in bulimia nervosa: a long-term follow-up study. Int J Eat Disord 51(12):1331–1338, 2018a 30520522

Frederiksen TC, Krogh Christiansen M, Charmoth Østergaard P, et al: QTc interval and risk of cardiac events in adults with anorexia nervosa: a long-term follow-up study. Circ Arrhythm Electrophysiol 11(8):e005995, 2018b 30030265

Frederiksen TC, Krogh Christiansen M, Clausen L, et al: Early repolarization pattern in adult females with eating disorders. Ann Noninvasive Electrocardiol 26(5):e12865, 2021 34114301

Freeman CP, Barry F, Dunkeld-Turnbull J, et al: Controlled trial of psychotherapy for bulimia nervosa. Br Med J (Clin Res Ed) 296(6621):521–525, 1988 3126890

Freeman R, Wieling W, Axelrod FB, et al: Consensus statement on the definition of orthostatic hypotension, neurally mediated syncope and the postural tachycardia syndrome. Auton Neurosci 161(1–2):46–48, 2011 21393070

Freizinger M, Jhe G, Pluhar E, et al: Integrating family based treatment principles in the acute inpatient treatment of adolescents with restrictive eating disorders. Psychol Res Behav Manag 14:449–454, 2021 33859508

Friederich H-C, Beate W, Zipfel S, et al: Anorexia Nervosa: Focal Psychodynamic Psychotherapy. Göttingen, Germany, Hogrefe, 2019

Frølich J, Winkler LA, Abrahamsen B, et al: Fractures in women with eating disorders: incidence, predictive factors, and the impact of disease remission: cohort study with background population controls. Int J Eat Disord 53(7):1080–1087, 2020 31922277

Froreich FV, Ratcliffe SE, Vartanian LR: Blind versus open weighing from an eating disorder patient perspective. J Eat Disord 8:39, 2020 32821384

Funk MC, Beach SR, Bostwick JR, et al: APA Resource Document: Resource Document on QTc Prolongation and Psychotropic Medications. Washington, DC, American Psychiatric Association, 2018

Fursland A, Watson HJ: Eating disorders: a hidden phenomenon in outpatient mental health? Int J Eat Disord 47(4):422–425, 2014 24136246

Gabel K, Pinhas L, Eisler I, et al: The effect of multiple family therapy on weight gain in adolescents with anorexia nervosa: pilot data. J Can Acad Child Adolesc Psychiatry 23(3):196–199, 2014 25320612

Galmiche M, Déchelotte P, Lambert G, et al: Prevalence of eating disorders over the 2000–2018 period: a systematic literature review. Am J Clin Nutr 109(5):1402–1413, 2019 31051507

Garber AK, Michihata N, Hetnal K, et al: A prospective examination of weight gain in hospitalized adolescents with anorexia nervosa on a recommended refeeding protocol. J Adolesc Health 50(1):24–29, 2012 22188830

Garber AK, Mauldin K, Michihata N, et al: Higher calorie diets increase rate of weight gain and shorten hospital stay in hospitalized adolescents with anorexia nervosa. J Adolesc Health 53(5):579–584, 2013 24054812

Garber AK, Sawyer SM, Golden NH, et al: A systematic review of approaches to refeeding in patients with anorexia nervosa. Int J Eat Disord 49(3):293–310, 2016 26661289

Garber AK, Cheng J, Accurso EC, et al: Weight loss and illness severity in adolescents with atypical anorexia nervosa. Pediatrics 144(6):e20192339, 2019 31694978

Garber AK, Cheng J, Accurso EC, et al: Short-term outcomes of the study of refeeding to optimize inpatient gains for patients with anorexia nervosa: a multicenter randomized clinical trial. JAMA Pediatr 175(1):19–27, 2021 33074282

Garcia FD, Grigioni S, Chelali S, et al: Validation of the French version of SCOFF questionnaire for screening of eating disorders among adults. World J Biol Psychiatry 11(7):888–893, 2010 20509759

Garcia-Campayo J, Sanz-Carrillo C, Ibañez JA, et al: Validation of the Spanish version of the SCOFF questionnaire for the screening of eating disorders in primary care. J Psychosom Res 59(2):51–55, 2005 16185998

Garner DM, Vitousek KM, Pike KM: Cognitive-behavioral therapy for anorexia nervosa, in Handbook of Treatment for Eating Disorders, 2nd Edition. Edited by Garner DM, Garfinkel PE. New York, Guilford, 1997

Garner DM, Anderson ML, Keiper CD, et al: Psychotropic medications in adult and adolescent eating disorders: clinical practice versus evidence-based recommendations. Eat Weight Disord 21(3):395–402, 2016 26830430

Gaudiani JL, Sabel AL, Mascolo M, et al: Severe anorexia nervosa: outcomes from a medical stabilization unit. Int J Eat Disord 45(1):85–92, 2012 22170021

Geist R, Heinmaa M, Stephens D, et al: Comparison of family therapy and family group psychoeducation in adolescents with anorexia nervosa. Can J Psychiatry 45(2):173–178, 2000 10742877

Gendall KA, Bulik CM, Joyce PR, et al: Menstrual cycle irregularity in bulimia nervosa: associated factors and changes with treatment. J Psychosom Res 49(6):409–415, 2000 11182433

George JB, Franko DL: Cultural issues in eating pathology and body image among children and adolescents. J Pediatr Psychol 35(3):231–242, 2010 19703916

Ghaderi A: Does individualization matter? A randomized trial of standardized (focused) versus individualized (broad) cognitive behavior therapy for bulimia nervosa. Behav Res Ther 44(2):273–288, 2006 16389065

Gianini L, Liu Y, Wang Y, et al: Abnormal eating behavior in video-recorded meals in anorexia nervosa. Eat Behav 19:28–32, 2015 26164671

Gibbings NK, Kurdyak PA, Colton PA, et al: Diabetic ketoacidosis and mortality in people with type 1 diabetes and eating disorders. Diabetes Care 44(8):1783–1787, 2021 34172488

Gibson D, Workman C, Mehler PS: Medical complications of anorexia nervosa and bulimia nervosa. Psychiatr Clin North Am 42(2):263–274, 2019 31046928

Gibson D, Watters A, Mehler PS: The intersect of gastrointestinal symptoms and malnutrition associated with anorexia nervosa and avoidant/restrictive food intake disorder: functional or pathophysiologic? A systematic review. Int J Eat Disord 54(6):1019–1054, 2021 34042203

Giovinazzo S, Sukkar SG, Rosa GM, et al: Anorexia nervosa and heart disease: a systematic review. Eat Weight Disord 24(2):199–207, 2019 30173377

Glasofer DR, Muratore AF, Attia E, et al: Predictors of illness course and health maintenance following inpatient treatment among patients with anorexia nervosa. J Eat Disord 8(1):69, 2020 33292619

Glisenti K, Strodl E, King R, et al: The feasibility of emotion-focused therapy for binge-eating disorder: a pilot randomised wait-list control trial. J Eat Disord 9(1):2, 2021 33407948

Godart N, Berthoz S, Curt F, et al: A randomized controlled trial of adjunctive family therapy and treatment as usual following inpatient treatment for anorexia nervosa adolescents. PLoS One 7(1):e28249, 2012 22238574

Golay A, Laurent-Jaccard A, Habicht F, et al: Effect of orlistat in obese patients with binge eating disorder. Obes Res 13(10):1701–1708, 2005 16286517

Goldberg HR, Katzman DK, Allen L, et al: The prevalence of children and adolescents at risk for avoidant restrictive food intake disorder in a pediatric and adolescent gynecology clinic. J Pediatr Adolesc Gynecol 33(5):466–469, 2020 32553711

Goldbloom DS, Olmsted MP: Pharmacotherapy of bulimia nervosa with fluoxetine: assessment of clinically significant attitudinal change. Am J Psychiatry 150(5):770–774, 1993 8480824

Goldbloom DS, Olmsted M, Davis R, et al: A randomized controlled trial of fluoxetine and cognitive behavioral therapy for bulimia nervosa: short-term outcome. Behav Res Ther 35(9):803–811, 1997 9299800

Golden NH, Jacobson MS, Schebendach J, et al: Resumption of menses in anorexia nervosa. Arch Pediatr Adolesc Med 151(1):16–21, 1997 9006523

Golden NH, Lanzkowsky L, Schebendach J, et al: The effect of estrogen-progestin treatment on bone mineral density in anorexia nervosa. J Pediatr Adolesc Gynecol 15(3):135–143, 2002 12106749

Golden NH, Iglesias EA, Jacobson MS, et al: Alendronate for the treatment of osteopenia in anorexia nervosa: a randomized, double-blind, placebo-controlled trial. J Clin Endocrinol Metab 90(6):3179–3185, 2005 15784715

Golden NH, Jacobson MS, Sterling WM, et al: Treatment goal weight in adolescents with anorexia nervosa: use of BMI percentiles. Int J Eat Disord 41(4):301–306, 2008 18176951

Golden NH, Keane-Miller C, Sainani KL, et al: Higher caloric intake in hospitalized adolescents with anorexia nervosa is associated with reduced length of stay and no increased rate of refeeding syndrome. J Adolesc Health 53(5):573–578, 2013 Erratum in J Adolesc Health 54(1):116, 2014

Golden NH, Abrams SA; Committee on Nutrition: Optimizing bone health in children and adolescents. Pediatrics 134(4):e1229–e1243, 2014 25266429

Golden NH, Katzman DK, Sawyer SM, et al: Position paper of the Society for Adolescent Health and Medicine: medical management of restrictive eating disorders in adolescents and young adults. J Adolesc Health 56(1):121–125, 2015a 25530605

Golden NH, Katzman DK, Sawyer SM, et al: Update on the medical management of eating disorders in adolescents. J Adolesc Health 56(4):370–375, 2015b 25659201

Golden NH, Cheng J, Kapphahn CJ, et al: Higher-calorie refeeding in anorexia nervosa: 1-year outcomes from a randomized controlled trial. Pediatrics 147(4):e2020037135, 2021 33753542

Goldstein DJ, Wilson MG, Thompson VL, et al: Long-term fluoxetine treatment of bulimia nervosa. Br J Psychiatry 166(5):660–666, 1995 7620754

Goldstein DJ, Wilson MG, Ascroft RC, et al: Effectiveness of fluoxetine therapy in bulimia nervosa regardless of comorbid depression. Int J Eat Disord 25(1):19–27, 1999 9924649

Gordon CM, Grace E, Emans SJ, et al: Effects of oral dehydroepiandrosterone on bone density in young women with anorexia nervosa: a randomized trial. J Clin Endocrinol Metab 87(11):4935–4941, 2002 12414853

Gordon CM, Zemel BS, Wren TA, et al: The determinants of peak bone mass. J Pediatr 180:261–269, 2017 27816219

Gorin AA, Le Grange D, Stone AA: Effectiveness of spouse involvement in cognitive behavioral therapy for binge eating disorder. Int J Eat Disord 33(4):421–433, 2003 12658672

Gorrell S, Loeb KL, Le Grange D: Family based treatment of eating disorders: a narrative review. Psychiatr Clin North Am 42(2):193–204, 2019 31046922

Gorwood P, Duriez P, Lengvenyte A, et al: Clinical insight in anorexia nervosa: associated and predictive factors. Psychiatry Res 281:112561, 2019 31521839

Gowers S, Norton K, Halek C, et al: Outcome of outpatient psychotherapy in a random allocation treatment study of anorexia nervosa. Int J Eat Disord 15(2):165–177, 1994 8173562

Gowers SG, Clark A, Roberts C, et al: Clinical effectiveness of treatments for anorexia nervosa in adolescents: randomised controlled trial. Br J Psychiatry 191:427–435, 2007 17978323

Gowers SG, Clark AF, Roberts C, et al: A randomised controlled multicentre trial of treatments for adolescent anorexia nervosa including assessment of cost-effectiveness and patient acceptability: the TOuCAN trial. Health Technol Assess 14(15):1–98, 2010 20334748

Grammer AC, Vázquez MM, Fitzsimmons-Craft EE, et al: Characterizing eating disorder diagnosis and related outcomes by sexual orientation and gender identity in a national sample of college students. Eat Behav 42:101528, 2021 34049053

Grant JE, Valle S, Cavic E, et al: A double-blind, placebo-controlled study of vortioxetine in the treatment of binge-eating disorder. Int J Eat Disord 52(7):786–794, 2019 30938842

Greenhalgh T, Robert G, Macfarlane F, et al: Diffusion of innovations in service organizations: systematic review and recommendations. Milbank Q 82(4):581–629, 2004 15595944

Grenon R, Schwartze D, Hammond N, et al: Group psychotherapy for eating disorders: a meta-analysis. Int J Eat Disord 50(9):997–1013, 2017 28771758

Griffiths RA, Hadzi-Pavlovic D, Channon-Little L: A controlled evaluation of hypnobehavioural treatment for bulimia nervosa: immediate pre-post treatment effects. Eur Eat Disord Rev 2(4):202–220, 1994

Griffiths RA, Hadzi-Pavlovic D, Channon-Little L: The short-term follow-up effects of hypnobehavioural and cognitive behavioural treatment for bulimia nervosa. Eur Eat Disord Rev 4(1):12–31, 1996

Grilo CM, Masheb RM: A randomized controlled comparison of guided self-help cognitive behavioral therapy and behavioral weight loss for binge eating disorder. Behav Res Ther 43(11):1509–1525, 2005 16159592

Grilo CM, Udo T: Examining the significance of age of onset in persons with lifetime anorexia nervosa: comparing child, adolescent, and emerging adult onsets in nationally representative U.S. study. Int J Eat Disord 54(9):1632–1640, 2021 34263464

Grilo CM, White MA: Orlistat with behavioral weight loss for obesity with versus without binge eating disorder: randomized placebo-controlled trial at a community mental health center serving educationally and economically disadvantaged Latino/as. Behav Res Ther 51(3):167–175, 2013 23376451

Grilo CM, Masheb RM, Salant SL: Cognitive behavioral therapy guided self-help and orlistat for the treatment of binge eating disorder: a randomized, double-blind, placebo-controlled trial. Biol Psychiatry 57(10):1193–1201, 2005a 15866560

Grilo CM, Masheb RM, Wilson GT: Efficacy of cognitive behavioral therapy and fluoxetine for the treatment of binge eating disorder: a randomized double-blind placebo-controlled comparison. Biol Psychiatry 57(3):301–309, 2005b 15691532

Grilo CM, Masheb RM, Wilson GT, et al: Cognitive-behavioral therapy, behavioral weight loss, and sequential treatment for obese patients with binge-eating disorder: a randomized controlled trial. J Consult Clin Psychol 79(5):675–685, 2011 21859185

Grilo CM, Crosby RD, White MA: Spanish-language Eating Disorder Examination interview: factor structure in Latino/as. Eat Behav 13(4):410–413, 2012a 23121800

Grilo CM, Crosby RD, Wilson GT, et al: 12-month follow-up of fluoxetine and cognitive behavioral therapy for binge eating disorder. J Consult Clin Psychol 80(6):1108–1113, 2012b 22985205

Grilo CM, White MA, Gueorguieva R, et al: Self-help for binge eating disorder in primary care: a randomized controlled trial with ethnically and racially diverse obese patients. Behav Res Ther 51(12):855–861, 2013 24189569

Grilo CM, Masheb RM, White MA, et al: Treatment of binge eating disorder in racially and ethnically diverse obese patients in primary care: randomized placebo-controlled clinical trial of self-help and medication. Behav Res Ther 58:1–9, 2014 24857821

Grilo CM, White MA, Ivezaj V, et al: Randomized controlled trial of behavioral weight loss and stepped care for binge-eating disorder: 12-month follow-up. Obesity (Silver Spring) 28(11):2116–2124, 2020a . 32985114

Grilo CM, White MA, Masheb RM, et al: Randomized controlled trial testing the effectiveness of adaptive "SMART" stepped-care treatment for adults with binge-eating disorder comorbid with obesity. Am Psychol 75(2):204–218, 2020b 32052995

Grinspoon S, Thomas L, Miller K, et al: Changes in regional fat redistribution and the effects of estrogen during spontaneous weight gain in women with anorexia nervosa. Am J Clin Nutr 73(5):865–869, 2001 11333838

Grinspoon S, Thomas L, Miller K, et al: Effects of recombinant human IGF-I and oral contraceptive administration on bone density in anorexia nervosa. J Clin Endocrinol Metab 87(6):2883–2891, 2002 12050268

Guarda AS, Wonderlich S, Kaye W, et al: A path to defining excellence in intensive treatment for eating disorders. Int J Eat Disord 51(9):1051–1055, 2018 30189103

Guerdjikova AI, McElroy SL, Kotwal R, et al: High-dose escitalopram in the treatment of binge-eating disorder with obesity: a placebo-controlled monotherapy trial. Hum Psychopharmacol 23(1):1–11, 2008 18058852

Guerdjikova AI, McElroy SL, Welge JA, et al: Lamotrigine in the treatment of binge-eating disorder with obesity: a randomized, placebo-controlled monotherapy trial. Int Clin Psychopharmacol 24(3):150–158, 2009 19357528

Guerdjikova AI, McElroy SL, Winstanley EL, et al: Duloxetine in the treatment of binge eating disorder with depressive disorders: a placebo-controlled trial. Int J Eat Disord 45(2):281–289, 2012 21744377

Guerdjikova AI, Mori N, Blom TJ, et al: Lisdexamfetamine dimesylate in binge eating disorder: a placebo controlled trial. Hum Psychopharmacol 31(5):382–391, 2016 27650406

Guinhut M, Melchior JC, Godart N, et al: Extremely severe anorexia nervosa: hospital course of 354 adult patients in a clinical nutrition-eating disorders-unit. Clin Nutr 40(4):1954–1965, 2021 33023762

Guyatt G, Gutterman D, Baumann MH, et al: Grading strength of recommendations and quality of evidence in clinical guidelines: report from an American College of Chest Physicians task force. Chest 129(1):174–181, 2006 16424429

Guyatt GH, Oxman AD, Kunz R, et al: Going from evidence to recommendations. BMJ 336(7652):1049–1051, 2008 18467413

Guyatt G, Eikelboom JW, Akl EA, et al: A guide to GRADE guidelines for the readers of JTH. J Thromb Haemost 11(8):1603–1608, 2013 23773710

Haas V, Kohn M, Körner T, et al: Practice-based evidence and clinical guidance to support accelerated re-nutrition of patients with anorexia nervosa. J Am Acad Child Adolesc Psychiatry 60(5):555–561, 2021 32998025

Habibzadeh N, Daneshmandi H: The effects of exercise in obese women with bulimia nervosa. Asian J Sports Med 1(4):209–213, 2010 22375209

Hackert AN, Kniskern MA, Beasley TM: Academy of Nutrition and Dietetics: revised 2020 standards of practice and standards of professional performance for registered dietitian nutritionists (competent, proficient, and expert) in eating disorders. J Acad Nutr Diet 120(11):1902–1919, 2020 33099403

Hagman J, Gralla J, Sigel E, et al: A double-blind, placebo-controlled study of risperidone for the treatment of adolescents and young adults with anorexia nervosa: a pilot study. J Am Acad Child Adolesc Psychiatry 50(9):915–924, 2011 21871373

Haines MS, Kimball A, Meenaghan E, et al: Sequential therapy with recombinant human igf-1 followed by risedronate increases spine bone mineral density in women with anorexia nervosa: a randomized, placebo-controlled trial. J Bone Miner Res 36(11):2116–2126, 2021 34355814

Hall A, Crisp AH: Brief psychotherapy in the treatment of anorexia nervosa: outcome at one year. Br J Psychiatry 151:185–191, 1987 3690108

Hall R, Keeble L, Sünram-Lea SI, To M: A review of risk factors associated with insulin omission for weight loss in type 1 diabetes. Clin Child Psychol Psychiatry 26(3):606–616, 2021 34121470

Halmi KA, Agras WS, Crow S, et al: Predictors of treatment acceptance and completion in anorexia nervosa: implications for future study designs. Arch Gen Psychiatry 62(7):776–781, 2005 15997019

Halvorsen I, Reas DL, Nilsen JV, et al: Naturalistic outcome of family based inpatient treatment for adolescents with anorexia nervosa. Eur Eat Disord Rev 26(2):141–145, 2018 29218761

Hamilton A, Mitchison D, Basten C, et al: Understanding treatment delay: perceived barriers preventing treatment-seeking for eating disorders. Aust N Z J Psychiatry 56(3):248–259, 2022 34250844

Hanachi M, Dicembre M, Rives-Lange C, et al: Micronutrients deficiencies in 374 severely malnourished anorexia nervosa inpatients. Nutrients 11(4):792, 2019 30959831

Hanachi M, Pleple A, Barry C, et al: Echocardiographic abnormalities in 124 severely malnourished adult anorexia nervosa patients: frequency and relationship with body composition and biological features. J Eat Disord 8(1):66, 2020 33292690

Harrer M, Adam SH, Messner EM, et al: Prevention of eating disorders at universities: a systematic review and meta-analysis. Int J Eat Disord 53(6):813–833, 2020 31943298

Harrop EN, Marlatt GA: The comorbidity of substance use disorders and eating disorders in women: prevalence, etiology, and treatment. Addict Behav 35(5):392–398, 2010 20074863

Harrop EN, Mensinger JL, Moore M, et al: Restrictive eating disorders in higher weight persons: a systematic review of atypical anorexia nervosa prevalence and consecutive admission literature. Int J Eat Disord 54(8):1328–1357, 2021 33864277

Hart LM, Wade T: Identifying research priorities in eating disorders: a Delphi study building consensus across clinicians, researchers, consumers, and carers in Australia. Int J Eat Disord 53(1):31–40, 2020 31571252

Hart S, Abraham S, Franklin RC, et al: Hypoglycaemia following a mixed meal in eating disorder patients. Postgrad Med J 87(1028):405–409, 2011 21389022

Haute Autorité de Santé: Clinical Practice Guidelines: Anorexia Nervosa: Management. Saint-Denis, France, 2010. Available at: https://www.has-sante.fr/upload/docs/application/pdf/2013-05/anorexia_nervosa_guidelines_2013-05-15_16-34-42_589.pdf. Accessed August 18, 2021.

Hay P, Chinn D, Forbes D, et al: Royal Australian and New Zealand College of Psychiatrists clinical practice guidelines for the treatment of eating disorders. Aust N Z J Psychiatry 48(11):977–1008, 2014 25351912

Hazlehurst JM, Armstrong MJ, Sherlock M, et al: A comparative quality assessment of evidence-based clinical guidelines in endocrinology. Clin Endocrinol (Oxf) 78(2):183–190, 2013 22624723

Hazzard VM, Bauer KW, Mukherjee B, et al: Associations between childhood maltreatment latent classes and eating disorder symptoms in a nationally representative sample of young adults in the United States. Child Abuse Negl 98:104171, 2019 31546098

Hazzard VM, Loth KA, Hooper L, et al: Food insecurity and eating disorders: a review of emerging evidence. Curr Psychiatry Rep 22(12):74, 2020 33125614

Hedges DW, Reimherr FW, Hoopes SP, et al: Treatment of bulimia nervosa with topiramate in a randomized, double-blind, placebo-controlled trial, part 2: improvement in psychiatric measures. J Clin Psychiatry 64(12):1449–1454, 2003 14728106

Hellner M, Bohon C, Kolander S, et al: Virtually delivered family based eating disorder treatment using an enhanced multidisciplinary care team: a case study. Clin Case Rep 9(6):e04173, 2021 34194768

Hemmingsen SD, Wesselhoeft R, Lichtenstein MB, et al: Cognitive improvement following weight gain in patients with anorexia nervosa: a systematic review. Eur Eat Disord Rev 29(3):402–426, 2021 33044043

Herman BK, Deal LS, DiBenedetti DB, et al: Development of the 7-Item Binge-Eating Disorder Screener (BEDS-7). Prim Care Companion CNS Disord 18(2):10.4088/PCC.15m01896, 2016 27486542

Herpertz S, Herpertz-Dahlmann B, Fichter M, et al: S3-leitlinie diagnostik und behandlung der essstörungen. German Society for Psychosomatic Medicine and Medical Psychotherapy, 2020. Available at: https://www.awmf.org/fileadmin/user_upload/Leitlinien/051_D-Ges_Psychosom_Med_u_aerztliche_Psychotherapie/051-026e_S3_eating-disorders-diagnosis-treatment_2020-07.pdf. Accessed September 13, 2021.

Herpertz-Dahlmann B, Schwarte R, Krei M, et al: Day-patient treatment after short inpatient care versus continued inpatient treatment in adolescents with anorexia nervosa (ANDI): a multicentre, randomised, open-label, non-inferiority trial. Lancet 383(9924):1222–1229, 2014 24439238

Herscovici CR, Kovalskys I, Orellana L: An exploratory evaluation of the family meal intervention for adolescent anorexia nervosa. Fam Process 56(2):364–375, 2017 26596997

Heruc G, Hart S, Stiles G, et al: ANZAED practice and training standards for dietitians providing eating disorder treatment. J Eat Disord 8(1):77, 2020 33317617

Hetterich L, Mack I, Giel KE, et al: An update on gastrointestinal disturbances in eating disorders. Mol Cell Endocrinol 497:110318, 2019 30359760

Hibbs R, Magill N, Goddard E, et al: Clinical effectiveness of a skills training intervention for caregivers in improving patient and caregiver health following in-patient treatment for severe anorexia nervosa: pragmatic randomised controlled trial. BJPsych Open 1(1):56–66, 2015 27703724

Hilbert A, Tuschen-Caffier B: Body image interventions in cognitive-behavioural therapy of binge-eating disorder: a component analysis. Behav Res Ther 42(11):1325–1339, 2004 15381441

Hilbert A, Bishop ME, Stein RI, et al: Long-term efficacy of psychological treatments for binge eating disorder. Br J Psychiatry 200(3):232–237, 2012 22282429

Hilbert A, Hoek HW, Schmidt R: Evidence-based clinical guidelines for eating disorders: international comparison. Curr Opin Psychiatry 30(6):423–437, 2017 28777107

Hilbert A, Petroff D, Herpertz S, et al: Meta-analysis of the efficacy of psychological and medical treatments for binge-eating disorder. J Consult Clin Psychol 87(1):91–105, 2019 30570304

Hildebrandt T, Michaelides A, Mackinnon D, et al: Randomized controlled trial comparing smartphone assisted versus traditional guided self-help for adults with binge eating. Int J Eat Disord 50(11):1313–1322, 2017 28960384

Hill DM, Craighead LW, Safer DL: Appetite-focused dialectical behavior therapy for the treatment of binge eating with purging: a preliminary trial. Int J Eat Disord 44(3):249–261, 2011 20196109

Himmerich H, Hotopf M, Shetty H, et al: Psychiatric comorbidity as a risk factor for mortality in people with anorexia nervosa. Eur Arch Psychiatry Clin Neurosci 269(3):351–359, 2019a 30120534

Himmerich H, Hotopf M, Shetty H, et al: Psychiatric comorbidity as a risk factor for the mortality of people with bulimia nervosa. Soc Psychiatry Psychiatr Epidemiol 54(7):813–821, 2019b 30756148

Hindley K, Fenton C, McIntosh J: A systematic review of enteral feeding by nasogastric tube in young people with eating disorders. J Eat Disord 9(1):90, 2021 34294163

Hodsoll J, Rhind C, Micali N, et al: A pilot, multicentre pragmatic randomised trial to explore the impact of carer skills training on carer and patient behaviours: testing the cognitive interpersonal model in adolescent anorexia nervosa. Eur Eat Disord Rev 25(6):551–561, 2017 28948663

Hooper L, Puhl R, Eisenberg ME, et al: Weight teasing experienced during adolescence and young adulthood: cross-sectional and longitudinal associations with disordered eating behaviors in an ethnically/racially and socioeconomically diverse sample. Int J Eat Disord 54(8):1449–1462, 2021 33969902

Hoopes SP, Reimherr FW, Hedges DW, et al: Treatment of bulimia nervosa with topiramate in a randomized, double-blind, placebo-controlled trial, part 1: improvement in binge and purge measures. J Clin Psychiatry 64(11):1335–1341, 2003 14658948

Hornberger LL, Lane MA, Committee on Adolescence: Identification and management of eating disorders in children and adolescents. Pediatrics 147(1):e2020040279, 2021. Available at: https://pediatrics.aappublications.org/content/pediatrics/147/1/e2020040279.full.pdf. Accessed August 24, 2021.

Horne RL, Ferguson JM, Pope HG Jr, et al: Treatment of bulimia with bupropion: a multicenter controlled trial. J Clin Psychiatry 49(7):262–266, 1988 3134343

Horvitz-Lennon M, Donohue JM, Domino ME, et al: Improving quality and diffusing best practices: the case of schizophrenia. Health Aff (Millwood) 28(3):701–712, 2009 19414878

Hower H, Reilly EE, Wierenga CE, et al: Last word: a call to view temperamental traits as dual vulnerabilities and strengths in anorexia nervosa. Eat Disord 29(2):1–10, 2021 33749529

Hsu LK, Clement L, Santhouse R, Ju ES: Treatment of bulimia nervosa with lithium carbonate: a controlled study. J Nerv Ment Dis 179(6):351–355, 1991 1904908

Hsu LK, Rand W, Sullivan S, et al: Cognitive therapy, nutritional therapy and their combination in the treatment of bulimia nervosa. Psychol Med 31(5):871–879, 2001 11459384

Hudson JI, McElroy SL, Raymond NC, et al: Fluvoxamine in the treatment of binge-eating disorder: a multicenter placebo-controlled, double-blind trial. Am J Psychiatry 155(12):1756–1762, 1998 9842788

Hudson JI, Hiripi E, Pope HG Jr, et al: The prevalence and correlates of eating disorders in the National Comorbidity Survey Replication. Biol Psychiatry 61(3):348–358, 2007 16815322

Hudson JI, McElroy SL, Ferreira-Cornwell MC, et al: Efficacy of lisdexamfetamine in adults with moderate to severe binge-eating disorder: a randomized clinical trial. JAMA Psychiatry 74(9):903–910, 2017 28700805

Huon GF: An initial validation of a self-help program for bulimia. Int J Eat Disord 4(4):573–588, 1985

Huryk KM, Casasnovas AF, Feehan M, et al: Lower rates of readmission following integration of family based treatment in a higher level of care. Eat Disord 29(6):677–684, 2021 33135596

Hütter G, Ganepola S, Hofmann WK: The hematology of anorexia nervosa. Int J Eat Disord 42(4):293–300, 2009 19040272

Imbierowicz K, Braks K, Jacoby GE, et al: High-caloric supplements in anorexia treatment. Int J Eat Disord 32(2):135–145, 2002 12210655

Institute of Medicine: Improving the Quality of Health Care for Mental and Substance-Use Conditions. Washington, DC, National Academies Press, 2006

Institute of Medicine: Clinical Practice Guidelines We Can Trust. Washington, DC, National Academies Press, 2011a

Institute of Medicine: Dietary Reference Intakes for Calcium and Vitamin D. Washington, DC, National Academies Press, 2011b

Institute of Medicine Committee on Quality of Health Care in America: Crossing the Quality Chasm: A New Health System for the 21st Century. Washington, DC, National Academies Press, 2001

International Association of Eating Disorders Professionals Foundation: The CEDRD in Eating Disorders Care. Pekin, IL, The International Association of Eating Disorders Professionals Foundation, 2017

Iwajomo T, Bondy SJ, de Oliveira C, et al: Excess mortality associated with eating disorders: population-based cohort study. Br J Psychiatry 219(3):487–493, 2021 33118892

Iyer SP, Spaeth-Rublee B, Pincus HA: Challenges in the operationalization of mental health quality measures: an assessment of alternatives. Psychiatr Serv 67(10):1057–1059, 2016 27301768

Jacobi C, Dahme B, Dittmann R: Cognitive-behavioural, fluoxetine and combined treatment for bulimia nervosa: short- and long-term results. Eur Eat Disord Rev 10(3):179–198, 2002

Jacobi C, Beintner I, Fittig E, et al: Web-based aftercare for women with bulimia nervosa following inpatient treatment: randomized controlled efficacy trial. J Med Internet Res 19(9):e321, 2017 28939544

Jackson JB, Pietrabissa G, Rossi A, et al: Brief strategic therapy and cognitive behavioral therapy for women with binge eating disorder and comorbid obesity: a randomized clinical trial one-year follow-up. J Consult Clin Psychol 86(8):688–701, 2018 30035585

Jäger B, Liedtke R, Künsebeck HW, et al: Psychotherapy and bulimia nervosa: evaluation and long-term follow-up of two conflict-orientated treatment conditions. Acta Psychiatr Scand 93(4):268–278, 1996 8712027

Jamieson A, Pelosi AJ: Use of denosumab in a patient with chronic anorexia nervosa and osteoporosis. Am J Med 129(2):e47, 2016 26777620

Javaras KN, Pope HG, Lalonde JK, et al: Co-occurrence of binge eating disorder with psychiatric and medical disorders. J Clin Psychiatry 69(2):266–273, 2008 18348600

Jenkins PE: Psychometric validation of the Clinical Impairment Assessment in a UK eating disorder service. Eat Behav 14(2):241–243, 2013 23557830

Jenkins PE: Cost-of-illness for non-underweight binge-eating disorders. Eat Weight Disord 27(4):1377–1384, 2022

Johnson KB, Neuss MJ, Detmer DE: Electronic health records and clinician burnout: a story of three eras. J Am Med Inform Assoc 28(5):967–973, 2021 33367815

Jones BA, Haycraft E, Bouman WP, et al: Risk factors for eating disorder psychopathology within the treatment seeking transgender population: the role of cross-sex hormone treatment. Eur Eat Disord Rev 26(2):120–128, 2018 29318711

Juarascio AS, Parker MN, Hunt R, et al: Mindfulness and acceptance-based behavioral treatment for bulimia-spectrum disorders: a pilot feasibility randomized trial. Int J Eat Disord 54(7):1270–1277, 2021 33851734

Kafantaris V, Leigh E, Hertz S, et al: A placebo-controlled pilot study of adjunctive olanzapine for adolescents with anorexia nervosa. J Child Adolesc Psychopharmacol 21(3):207–212, 2011 21663423

Kambanis PE, Kuhnle MC, Wons OB, et al: Prevalence and correlates of psychiatric comorbidities in children and adolescents with full and subthreshold avoidant/restrictive food intake disorder. Int J Eat Disord 53(2):256–265, 2020 31702051

Kamody RC, Grilo CM, Udo T: Disparities in DSM-5 defined eating disorders by sexual orientation among U.S. adults. Int J Eat Disord 53(2):278–287, 2020 31670848

Kanerva R, Rissanen A, Sarna S: Fluoxetine in the treatment of anxiety, depressive symptoms, and eating-related symptoms in bulimia nervosa. Nord J Psychiatry 49(4):237–242, 1995

Karam AM, Fitzsimmons-Craft EE, Tanofsky-Kraff M, et al: Interpersonal psychotherapy and the treatment of eating disorders. Psychiatr Clin North Am 42(2):205–218, 2019 31046923

Kask J, Ekselius L, Brandt L, et al: Mortality in women with anorexia nervosa: the role of comorbid psychiatric disorders. Psychosom Med 78(8):910–919, 2016 27136502

Kask J, Ramklint M, Kolia N, et al: Anorexia nervosa in males: excess mortality and psychiatric co-morbidity in 609 Swedish in-patients. Psychol Med 47(8):1489–1499, 2017 28162109

Katzman MA, Bara-Carril N, Rabe-Hesketh S, et al: A randomized controlled two-stage trial in the treatment of bulimia nervosa, comparing CBT versus motivational enhancement in Phase 1 followed by group versus individual CBT in Phase 2. Psychosom Med 72(7):656–663, 2010 20668284

Katzman DK, Spettigue W, Agostino H, et al: Incidence and age- and sex-specific differences in the clinical presentation of children and adolescents with avoidant restrictive food intake disorder. JAMA Pediatr 175(12):e213861, 2021 34633419

Kaye WH, Nagata T, Weltzin TE, et al: Double-blind placebo-controlled administration of fluoxetine in restricting- and restricting-purging-type anorexia nervosa. Biol Psychiatry 49(7):644–652, 2001 11297722

Kazdin AE, Fitzsimmons-Craft EE, Wilfley DE: Addressing critical gaps in the treatment of eating disorders. Int J Eat Disord 50(3):170–189, 2017 28102908

Keel PK, Mitchell JE, Davis TL, Crow SJ: Long-term impact of treatment in women diagnosed with bulimia nervosa. Int J Eat Disord 31(2):151–158, 2002 11920976

Keery H, LeMay-Russell S, Barnes TL, et al: Attributes of children and adolescents with avoidant/restrictive food intake disorder. J Eat Disord 7:31, 2019 31528341

Keshishian AC, Tabri N, Becker KR, et al: Eating disorder recovery is associated with absence of major depressive disorder and substance use disorders at 22-year longitudinal follow-up. Compr Psychiatry 90:49–51, 2019 30685636

Keski-Rahkonen A: Epidemiology of binge eating disorder: prevalence, course, comorbidity, and risk factors. Curr Opin Psychiatry 34(6):525–531, 2021 34494972

Kesztyüs D, Lampl J, Kesztyüs T: The weight problem: overview of the most common concepts for body mass and fat distribution and critical consideration of their usefulness for risk assessment and practice. Int J Environ Res Public Health 18(21):11070, 2021 34769593

Keys A, Brozek J, Henshel A, et al: The Biology of Human Starvation, Vols 1–2. Minneapolis, MN, University of Minnesota Press, 1950

Khosla S, Monroe DG: Regulation of bone metabolism by sex steroids. Cold Spring Harb Perspect Med 8(1):a031211, 2018 28710257

Kimber M, McTavish JR, Couturier J, et al: Consequences of child emotional abuse, emotional neglect and exposure to intimate partner violence for eating disorders: a systematic critical review. BMC Psychol 5(1):33, 2017 28938897

Kinzig KP, Coughlin JW, Redgrave GW, et al: Insulin, glucose, and pancreatic polypeptide responses to a test meal in restricting type anorexia nervosa before and after weight restoration. Am J Physiol Endocrinol Metab 292(5):E1441–E1446, 2007 17264227

Klein AS, Skinner JB, Hawley KM: Targeting binge eating through components of dialectical behavior therapy: preliminary outcomes for individually supported diary card self-monitoring versus group-based DBT. Psychotherapy (Chic) 50(4):543–552, 2013 24295464

Klibanski A, Biller BM, Schoenfeld DA, et al: The effects of estrogen administration on trabecular bone loss in young women with anorexia nervosa. J Clin Endocrinol Metab 80(3):898–904, 1995 7883849

Kliem S, Schmidt R, Vogel M, et al: An 8-item short form of the Eating Disorder Examination-Questionnaire adapted for children (ChEDE-Q8). Int J Eat Disord 50(6):679–686, 2017 28122128

Knatz Peck S, Towne T, Wierenga CE, et al: Temperament-based treatment for young adults with eating disorders: acceptability and initial efficacy of an intensive, multi-family, parent-involved treatment. J Eat Disord 9(1):110, 2021 34496951

Konstantakopoulos G, Tchanturia K, Surguladze SA, et al: Insight in eating disorders: clinical and cognitive correlates. Psychol Med 41(9):1951–1961, 2011 21211101

Konstantakopoulos G, Georgantopoulos G, Gonidakis F, et al: Development and validation of the Schedule for the Assessment of Insight in Eating Disorders (SAI-ED). Psychiatry Res 292:113308, 2020 32707219

Kostro K, Lerman JB, Attia E: The current status of suicide and self-injury in eating disorders: a narrative review. J Eat Disord 2:19, 2014 26034603

Krahn DD, Rock C, Dechert RE, et al: Changes in resting energy expenditure and body composition in anorexia nervosa patients during refeeding. J Am Diet Assoc 93(4):434–438, 1993 8454812

Krantz MJ, Blalock DV, Tanganyika K, et al: Is QTc-interval prolongation an inherent feature of eating disorders? A cohort Study. Am J Med 133(9):1088–1094, 2020 32165189

Kristeller J, Wolever RQ, Sheets V: Mindfulness-based eating awareness training (mb-eat) for binge eating: a randomized clinical trial. Mindfulness 5(3):282–297, 2014

Kröger C, Schweiger U, Sipos V, et al: Dialectical behaviour therapy and an added cognitive behavioural treatment module for eating disorders in women with borderline personality disorder and anorexia nervosa or bulimia nervosa who failed to respond to previous treatments: an open trial with a 15-month follow-up. J Behav Ther Exp Psychiatry 41(4):381–388, 2010 20444442

Krug I, Treasure J, Anderluh M, et al: Present and lifetime comorbidity of tobacco, alcohol and drug use in eating disorders: a European multicenter study. Drug Alcohol Depend 97(1–2):169–179, 2008 18571341

Kutz AM, Marsh AG, Gunderson CG, et al: Eating disorder screening: a systematic review and meta-analysis of diagnostic test characteristics of the SCOFF. J Gen Intern Med 35(3):885–893, 2020 31705473

Laederach-Hofmann K, Graf C, Horber F, et al: Imipramine and diet counseling with psychological support in the treatment of obese binge eaters: a randomized, placebo-controlled double-blind study. Int J Eat Disord 26(3):231–244, 1999 10441239

Lammers MW, Vroling MS, Crosby RD, et al: Dialectical behavior therapy adapted for binge eating compared to cognitive behavior therapy in obese adults with binge eating disorder: a controlled study. J Eat Disord 8:27, 2020

Lavender JM, Brown TA, Murray SB: Men, muscles, and eating disorders: an overview of traditional and muscularity-oriented disordered eating. Curr Psychiatry Rep 19(6):32, 2017 28470486

Le Grange D: Family therapy for adolescent anorexia nervosa. J Clin Psychol 55(6):727–739, 1999 10445863

Le Grange D, Gorin A, Dymek M, et al: Does ecological momentary assessment improve cognitive behavioural therapy for binge eating disorder? A pilot study. Eur Eat Disord Rev 10(5):316–328, 2002

Le Grange D, Crosby RD, Rathouz PJ, et al: A randomized controlled comparison of family based treatment and supportive psychotherapy for adolescent bulimia nervosa. Arch Gen Psychiatry 64(9):1049–1056, 2007 17768270

Le Grange D, Accurso EC, Lock J, et al: Early weight gain predicts outcome in two treatments for adolescent anorexia nervosa. Int J Eat Disord 47(2):124–129, 2014a 24190844

Le Grange D, Lock J, Accurso EC, et al: Relapse from remission at two- to four-year follow-up in two treatments for adolescent anorexia nervosa. J Am Acad Child Adolesc Psychiatry 53(11):1162–1167, 2014b 25440306

Le Grange D, Lock J, Agras WS, et al: Randomized clinical trial of family based treatment and cognitive-behavioral therapy for adolescent bulimia nervosa. J Am Acad Child Adolesc Psychiatry 54(11):886–894, 2015 26506579

Le Grange D, Hughes EK, Court A, et al: Randomized clinical trial of parent-focused treatment and family based treatment for adolescent anorexia nervosa. J Am Acad Child Adolesc Psychiatry 55(8):683–692, 2016 27453082

Le Grange D, Eckhardt S, Dalle Grave R, et al: Enhanced cognitive-behavior therapy and family based treatment for adolescents with an eating disorder: a non-randomized effectiveness trial. Psychol Med December 3, 2020 33267919 Epub ahead of print

Lebow J, Sim LA, Kransdorf LN: Prevalence of a history of overweight and obesity in adolescents with restrictive eating disorders. J Adolesc Health 56(1):19–24, 2015 25049202

Lebwohl B, Haggård L, Emilsson L, et al: Psychiatric disorders in patients with a diagnosis of celiac disease during childhood from 1973 to 2016. Clin Gastroenterol Hepatol 19(10):2093–2101, 2021 32801012

Lee DH, Keum N, Hu FB, et al: Development and validation of anthropometric prediction equations for lean body mass, fat mass and percent fat in adults using the National Health and Nutrition Examination Survey (NHANES) 1999–2006. Br J Nutr 118(10):858–866, 2017 29110742

Legg NK, Turner BJ: Personality correlates of eating pathology severity and subtypes in The National Comorbidity Survey Adolescent Supplement. J Clin Psychol 77(1):189–210, 2021 32627202

Leitenberg H, Rosen JC, Gross J, et al: Exposure plus response-prevention treatment of bulimia nervosa. J Consult Clin Psychol 56(4):535–541, 1988 3198810

Leombruni P, Amianto F, Delsedime N, et al: Citalopram versus fluoxetine for the treatment of patients with bulimia nervosa: a single-blind randomized controlled trial. Adv Ther 23(3):481–494, 2006 16912031

Leombruni P, Pierò A, Lavagnino L, et al: A randomized, double-blind trial comparing sertraline and fluoxetine 6-month treatment in obese patients with binge eating disorder. Prog Neuropsychopharmacol Biol Psychiatry 32(6):1599–1605, 2008 18598735

Levinson CA, Spoor SP, Keshishian AC, et al: Pilot outcomes from a multidisciplinary telehealth versus in-person intensive outpatient program for eating disorders during versus before the Covid-19 pandemic. Int J Eat Disord 54(9):1672–1679, 2021 34245028

Lewer M, Kosfelder J, Michalak J, et al: Effects of a cognitive-behavioral exposure-based body image therapy for overweight females with binge eating disorder: a pilot study. J Eat Disord 5:43, 2017 29296280

Lexicomp: Lexicomp Database. Riverwoods IL, Wolters Kluwer Health, 2021

Lichtenstein MB, Haastrup L, Johansen KK, et al: Validation of the eating disorder examination questionnaire in Danish eating disorder patients and athletes. J Clin Med 10(17):3976, 2021 34501422

Lie SØ, Rø Ø, Bang L: Is bullying and teasing associated with eating disorders? A systematic review and meta-analysis. Int J Eat Disord 52(5):497–514, 2019 30706957

Lie SØ, Bulik CM, Andreassen OA, et al: Stressful life events among individuals with a history of eating disorders: a case-control comparison. BMC Psychiatry 21(1):501, 2021a 34645394

Lie SØ, Bulik CM, Andreassen OA, et al: The association between bullying and eating disorders: a case-control study. Int J Eat Disord 54(8):1405–1414, 2021b 33942329

Lilenfeld LR, Wonderlich S, Riso LP, et al: Eating disorders and personality: a methodological and empirical review. Clin Psychol Rev 26(3):299–320, 2006 16330138

Lin JA, Hartman-Munick SM, Kells MR, et al: The impact of the COVID-19 pandemic on the number of adolescents/young adults seeking eating disorder-related care. J Adolesc Health 69(4):660–663, 2021 34266715

Linardon J, Shatte A, Messer M, et al: E-mental health interventions for the treatment and prevention of eating disorders: an updated systematic review and meta-analysis. J Consult Clin Psychol 88(11):994–1007, 2020 32852971

Liu B, Du Y, Wu Y, et al: Trends in obesity and adiposity measures by race or ethnicity among adults in the United States 2011–18: population based study. BMJ 372(365):n365, 2021 33727242

Lock J, Le Grange D: Treatment Manual for Anorexia Nervosa: A Family Based Approach, 2nd Edition. New York, Guilford, 2013

Lock J, Agras WS, Bryson S, et al: A comparison of short- and long-term family therapy for adolescent anorexia nervosa. J Am Acad Child Adolesc Psychiatry 44(7):632–639, 2005 15968231

Lock J, Couturier J, Agras WS: Comparison of long-term outcomes in adolescents with anorexia nervosa treated with family therapy. J Am Acad Child Adolesc Psychiatry 45(6):666–672, 2006a 16721316

Lock J, Couturier J, Bryson S, et al: Predictors of dropout and remission in family therapy for adolescent anorexia nervosa in a randomized clinical trial. Int J Eat Disord 39(8):639–647, 2006b 16927385

Lock J, Le Grange D, Agras WS, et al: Randomized clinical trial comparing family based treatment with adolescent-focused individual therapy for adolescents with anorexia nervosa. Arch Gen Psychiatry 67(10):1025–1032, 2010 20921118

Lock J, Agras WS, Fitzpatrick KK, et al: Is outpatient cognitive remediation therapy feasible to use in randomized clinical trials for anorexia nervosa? Int J Eat Disord 46(6):567–575, 2013 23625628

Lock J, La Via MC; American Academy of Child and Adolescent Psychiatry Committee on Quality Issues: Practice parameter for the assessment and treatment of children and adolescents with eating disorders. J Am Acad Child Adolesc Psychiatry 54(5):412–425, 2015a 25901778

Lock J, Le Grange D, Agras WS, et al: Can adaptive treatment improve outcomes in family based therapy for adolescents with anorexia nervosa? Feasibility and treatment effects of a multi-site treatment study. Behav Res Ther 73:90–95, 2015b 26276704

Lock J, Agras WS, Bryson SW, et al: Does family based treatment reduce the need for hospitalization in adolescent anorexia nervosa? Int J Eat Disord 49(9):891–894, 2016 27062400

Lock J, Fitzpatrick KK, Agras WS, et al: Feasibility study combining art therapy or cognitive remediation therapy with family based treatment for adolescent anorexia nervosa. Eur Eat Disord Rev 26(1):62–68, 2018 29152825

Lock J, Sadeh-Sharvit S, L'Insalata A: Feasibility of conducting a randomized clinical trial using family based treatment for avoidant/restrictive food intake disorder. Int J Eat Disord 52(6):746–751, 2019 30924958

Lock J, Couturier J, Matheson BE, et al: Feasibility of conducting a randomized controlled trial comparing family based treatment via videoconferencing and online guided self-help family based treatment for adolescent anorexia nervosa. Int J Eat Disord 54(11):1998–2008, 2021 34553395

Loeb KL, Wilson GT, Gilbert JS, et al: Guided and unguided self-help for binge eating. Behav Res Ther 38(3):259–272, 2000 10665159

Lucas AR, Melton LJ 3rd, Crowson CS, et al: Long-term fracture risk among women with anorexia nervosa: a population-based cohort study. Mayo Clin Proc 74(10):972–977, 1999 10918862

Lund BC, Hernandez ER, Yates WR, et al: Rate of inpatient weight restoration predicts outcome in anorexia nervosa. Int J Eat Disord 42(4):301–305, 2009 19107835

Lydecker JA, Grilo CM: Fathers and mothers with eating-disorder psychopathology: associations with child eating-disorder behaviors. J Psychosom Res 86:63–69, 2016 27302549

Lydecker JA, Grilo CM: Psychiatric comorbidity as predictor and moderator of binge-eating disorder treatment outcomes: an analysis of aggregated randomized controlled trials. Psychol Med April 14, 2021 33849682 Epub ahead of print

Madden S, Miskovic-Wheatley J, Wallis A, et al: A randomized controlled trial of in-patient treatment for anorexia nervosa in medically unstable adolescents. Psychol Med 45(2):415–427, 2015 25017941

Madowitz J, Matheson BE, Liang J: The relationship between eating disorders and sexual trauma. Eat Weight Disord 20(3):281–293, 2015 25976911

Magill N, Rhind C, Hibbs R, et al: Two-year follow-up of a pragmatic randomised controlled trial examining the effect of adding a carer's skill training intervention in inpatients with anorexia nervosa. Eur Eat Disord Rev 24(2):122–130, 2016 26695507

Maguen S, Hebenstreit C, Li Y, et al: Screen for Disordered Eating: improving the accuracy of eating disorder screening in primary care. Gen Hosp Psychiatry 50:20–25, 2018 28987918

Mahr F, Billman M, Essayli JH, et al: Selective serotonin reuptake inhibitors and hydroxyzine in the treatment of avoidant/restrictive food intake disorder in children and adolescents: rationale and evidence. J Child Adolesc Psychopharmacol 32(2):117–121, 2021 34619050

Makino M, Tsuboi K, Dennerstein L: Prevalence of eating disorders: a comparison of Western and non-Western countries. MedGenMed 6(3):49, 2004 15520673

Maraldo TM, Fewell L, Vander Wal JS: Factor structure and psychometric properties of the Clinical Impairment Assessment 3.0 (CIA) in a clinical eating disorder sample. Eat Behav 40:101469, 2021 33418485

Mårild K, Størdal K, Bulik CM, et al: Celiac disease and anorexia nervosa: a nationwide study. Pediatrics 139(5):e20164367, 2017 28557761

Marion M, Lacroix S, Caquard M, et al: Earlier diagnosis in anorexia nervosa: better watch growth charts! J Eat Disord 8:42, 2020 32905240

Marques L, Alegria M, Becker AE, et al: Comparative prevalence, correlates of impairment, and service utilization for eating disorders across US ethnic groups: implications for reducing ethnic disparities in health care access for eating disorders. Int J Eat Disord 44(5):412–420, 2011 20665700

Martín J, Padierna A, Unzurrunzaga A, et al: Adaptation and validation of the Spanish version of the Clinical Impairment Assessment Questionnaire. Appetite 91:20–27, 2015 25839732

Masheb RM, Grilo CM, Rolls BJ: A randomized controlled trial for obesity and binge eating disorder: low-energy-density dietary counseling and cognitive-behavioral therapy. Behav Res Ther 49(12):821–829, 2011 22005587

Mason TB, Tackett AP, Smith CE, et al: Tobacco product use for weight control as an eating disorder behavior: recommendations for future clinical and public health research. Int J Eat Disord 55(3):313–317, 2021 34866222

Matheson BE, Bohon C, Lock J: Family based treatment via videoconference: clinical recommendations for treatment providers during COVID-19 and beyond. Int J Eat Disord 53(7):1142–1154, 2020 32533799

McCann UD, Agras WS: Successful treatment of nonpurging bulimia nervosa with desipramine: a double-blind, placebo-controlled study. Am J Psychiatry 147(11):1509–1513, 1990 2221164

McElroy SL, Arnold LM, Shapira NA, et al: Topiramate in the treatment of binge eating disorder associated with obesity: a randomized, placebo-controlled trial. Am J Psychiatry 160(2):255–261, 2003 12562571

McElroy SL, Kotwal R, Guerdjikova AI, et al: Zonisamide in the treatment of binge eating disorder with obesity: a randomized controlled trial. J Clin Psychiatry 67(12):1897–1906, 2006 17194267

McElroy SL, Guerdjikova A, Kotwal R, et al: Atomoxetine in the treatment of binge-eating disorder: a randomized placebo-controlled trial. J Clin Psychiatry 68(3):390–398, 2007a 17388708

McElroy SL, Hudson JI, Capece JA, et al: Topiramate for the treatment of binge eating disorder associated with obesity: a placebo-controlled study. Biol Psychiatry 61(9):1039–1048, 2007b 17258690

McElroy SL, Guerdjikova AI, Winstanley EL, et al: Acamprosate in the treatment of binge eating disorder: a placebo-controlled trial. Int J Eat Disord 44(1):81–90, 2011 21080416

McElroy SL, Guerdjikova AI, Mori N, et al: Armodafinil in binge eating disorder: a randomized, placebo-controlled trial. Int Clin Psychopharmacol 30(4):209–215, 2015a 26011779

McElroy SL, Hudson JI, Mitchell JE, et al: Efficacy and safety of lisdexamfetamine for treatment of adults with moderate to severe binge-eating disorder: a randomized clinical trial. JAMA Psychiatry 72(3):235–246, 2015b 25587645

McElroy SL, Hudson J, Ferreira-Cornwell MC, et al: Lisdexamfetamine dimesylate for adults with moderate to severe binge eating disorder: results of two pivotal phase 3 randomized controlled trials. Neuropsychopharmacology 41(5):1251–1260, 2016a 26346638

McElroy SL, Mitchell JE, Wilfley D, et al: Lisdexamfetamine dimesylate effects on binge eating behaviour and obsessive-compulsive and impulsive features in adults with binge eating disorder. Eur Eat Disord Rev 24(3):223–231, 2016b 26621156

McElroy SL, Hudson JI, Gasior M, et al: Time course of the effects of lisdexamfetamine dimesylate in two phase 3, randomized, double-blind, placebo-controlled trials in adults with binge-eating disorder. Int J Eat Disord 50(8):884–892, 2017 28481434

McGuinness LA, Higgins JPT: Risk-of-bias VISualization (robvis): an R package and Shiny web app for visualizing risk-of-bias assessments. Res Syn Meth 12(1):55–61, 2020 32336025

McIntosh VV, Jordan J, Carter FA, et al: Three psychotherapies for anorexia nervosa: a randomized, controlled trial. Am J Psychiatry 162(4):741–747, 2005 15800147

McIntosh VV, Jordan J, Luty SE, et al: Specialist supportive clinical management for anorexia nervosa. Int J Eat Disord 39(8):625–632, 2006 16937382

McIntosh VVW, Jordan J, Carter JD, et al: Psychotherapy for transdiagnostic binge eating: a randomized controlled trial of cognitive-behavioural therapy, appetite-focused cognitive-behavioural therapy, and schema therapy. Psychiatry Res 240:412–420, 2016 27149410

Meurman JH, ten Cate JM: Pathogenesis and modifying factors of dental erosion. Eur J Oral Sci 104(2 Pt 2):199–206, 1996 8804887

Michihata N, Matsui H, Fushimi K, et al: Comparison between enteral nutrition and intravenous hyperalimentation in patients with eating disorders: results from the Japanese diagnosis procedure combination database. Eat Weight Disord 19(4):473–478, 2014 25150426

Milano W, Petrella C, Sabatino C, et al: Treatment of bulimia nervosa with sertraline: a randomized controlled trial. Adv Ther 21(4):232–237, 2004 15605617

Milano W, Petrella C, Capasso A: Treatment of bulimia nervosa with citalopram: a randomized controlled trial. Biomed Res 16(2):85–87, 2005

Milano W, De Rosa M, Milano L, et al: A comparative study between three different SSRIs in the treatment of bulimia nervosa. Curr Neurobiol 4(1–2):39–42, 2013

Miller KK, Grinspoon SK, Ciampa J, et al: Medical findings in outpatients with anorexia nervosa. Arch Intern Med 165(5):561–566, 2005 15767533

Miller KK, Meenaghan E, Lawson EA, et al: Effects of risedronate and low-dose transdermal testosterone on bone mineral density in women with anorexia nervosa: a randomized, placebo-controlled study. J Clin Endocrinol Metab 96(7):2081–2088, 2011 21525157

Misra M, Klibanski A: Endocrine consequences of anorexia nervosa. Lancet Diabetes Endocrinol 2(7):581–592, 2014 24731664

Misra M, Katzman DK, Cord J, et al: Bone metabolism in adolescent boys with anorexia nervosa. J Clin Endocrinol Metab 93(8):3029–3036, 2008a 18544623

Misra M, Prabhakaran R, Miller KK, et al: Weight gain and restoration of menses as predictors of bone mineral density change in adolescent girls with anorexia nervosa-1. J Clin Endocrinol Metab 93(4):1231–1237, 2008b 18089702

Misra M, Katzman D, Miller KK, et al: Physiologic estrogen replacement increases bone density in adolescent girls with anorexia nervosa. J Bone Miner Res 26(10):2430–2438, 2011 21698665

Misra M, Katzman DK, Estella NM, et al: Impact of physiologic estrogen replacement on anxiety symptoms, body shape perception, and eating attitudes in adolescent girls with anorexia nervosa: data from a randomized controlled trial. J Clin Psychiatry 74(8):e765–e771, 2013 24021517

Misra M, Golden NH, Katzman DK: State of the art systematic review of bone disease in anorexia nervosa. Int J Eat Disord 49(3):276–292, 2016 26311400

Mitchell JE: Medical comorbidity and medical complications associated with binge-eating disorder. Int J Eat Disord 49(3):319–323, 2016 26311499

Mitchell JE, Groat R: A placebo-controlled, double-blind trial of amitriptyline in bulimia. J Clin Psychopharmacol 4(4):186–193, 1984 6381556

Mitchell JE, Pyle RL, Eckert ED, et al: A comparison study of antidepressants and structured intensive group psychotherapy in the treatment of bulimia nervosa. Arch Gen Psychiatry 47(2):149–157, 1990 2405806

Mitchell JE, Pyle RL, Pomeroy C, et al: Cognitive-behavioral group psychotherapy of bulimia nervosa: importance of logistical variables. Int J Eat Disord 14(3):277–287, 1993 8275064

Mitchell JE, Fletcher L, Hanson K, et al: The relative efficacy of fluoxetine and manual-based self-help in the treatment of outpatients with bulimia nervosa. J Clin Psychopharmacol 21(3):298–304, 2001 11386493

Mitchell JE, Halmi K, Wilson GT, et al: A randomized secondary treatment study of women with bulimia nervosa who fail to respond to CBT. Int J Eat Disord 32(3):271–281, 2002 12210641

Mitchell JE, Crosby RD, Wonderlich SA, et al: A randomized trial comparing the efficacy of cognitive-behavioral therapy for bulimia nervosa delivered via telemedicine versus face-to-face. Behav Res Ther 46(5):581–592, 2008 18374304

Mitchell JE, Agras S, Crow S, et al: Stepped care and cognitive-behavioural therapy for bulimia nervosa: randomised trial. Br J Psychiatry 198(5):391–397, 2011 21415046

Modan-Moses D, Yaroslavsky A, Novikov I, et al: Stunting of growth as a major feature of anorexia nervosa in male adolescents. Pediatrics 111(2):270–276, 2003 12563050

Modan-Moses D, Yaroslavsky A, Pinhas-Hamiel O, et al: Prospective longitudinal assessment of linear growth and adult height in female adolescents with anorexia nervosa. J Clin Endocrinol Metab 106(1):e1–e10, 2021 32816013

Molendijk ML, Hoek HW, Brewerton TD, et al: Childhood maltreatment and eating disorder pathology: a systematic review and dose-response meta-analysis. Psychol Med 47(8):1–15, 2017 28100288

Mond JM, Hay PJ, Rodgers B, et al: Validity of the Eating Disorder Examination Questionnaire (EDE-Q) in screening for eating disorders in community samples. Behav Res Ther 42(5):551–567, 2004 15033501

Monge MC, Forman SF, McKenzie NM, et al: Use of psychopharmacologic medications in adolescents with restrictive eating disorders: analysis of data from the National Eating Disorder Quality Improvement Collaborative. J Adolesc Health 57(1):66–72, 2015 26095410

Monteleone AM, Cascino G, Ruzzi V, et al: Multiple levels assessment of the RDoC "system for social process" in eating disorders: biological, emotional and cognitive responses to the Trier Social Stress Test. J Psychiatr Res 130:160–166, 2020 32823049

Morgan JF, Reid F, Lacey JH: The SCOFF questionnaire: assessment of a new screening tool for eating disorders. BMJ 319(7223):1467–1468, 1999 10582927

Mosekilde L, Vestergaard P, Rejnmark L: The pathogenesis, treatment and prevention of osteoporosis in men. Drugs 73(1):15–29, 2013 23329464

Mountford VA, Brown A, Bamford B, et al: BodyWise: evaluating a pilot body image group for patients with anorexia nervosa. Eur Eat Disord Rev 23(1):62–67, 2015 25382845

Munsch S, Biedert E, Meyer A, et al: A randomized comparison of cognitive behavioral therapy and behavioral weight loss treatment for overweight individuals with binge eating disorder. Int J Eat Disord 40(2):102–113, 2007 17089420

Munsch S, Meyer AH, Biedert E: Efficacy and predictors of long-term treatment success for cognitive-behavioral treatment and behavioral weight-loss-treatment in overweight individuals with binge eating disorder. Behav Res Ther 50(12):775–785, 2012 23099111

Murphy R, Straebler S, Basden S, et al: Interpersonal psychotherapy for eating disorders. Clin Psychol Psychother 19(2):150–158, 2012 22362599

Murray HB, Rao FU, Baker C, et al: Prevalence and characteristics of avoidant/restrictive food intake disorder in pediatric neurogastroenterology patients. J Pediatr Gastroenterol Nutr 18(9):1995–2002, 2021 31669056

Nagata JM, Golden NH, Leonard MB, et al: Assessment of sex differences in fracture risk among patients with anorexia nervosa: a population-based cohort study using the Health Improvement Network. J Bone Miner Res 32(5):1082–1089, 2017 28019700

Nagata JM, Compte EJ, Cattle CJ, et al: Community norms for the Eating Disorder Examination Questionnaire (EDE-Q) among gender-expansive populations. J Eat Disord 8(1):74, 2020a 33292636

Nagata JM, Ganson KT, Austin SB: Emerging trends in eating disorders among sexual and gender minorities. Curr Opin Psychiatry 33(6):562–567, 2020b 32858597

Nagata JM, Murray SB, Compte EJ, et al: Community norms for the Eating Disorder Examination Questionnaire (EDE-Q) among transgender men and women. Eat Behav 37:101381, 2020c 32416588

Nakahara T, Nagai N, Tanaka M, et al: The effects of bone therapy on tibial bone loss in young women with anorexia nervosa. Int J Eat Disord 39(1):20–26, 2006 16231362

National Guideline Alliance (UK): Eating Disorders: Recognition and Treatment. London, National Institute for Health and Care Excellence (UK), 2020

Nauta H, Hospers G, Jansen A: A comparison between a cognitive and a behavioral treatment for obese binge eaters and obese non-binge eaters. Behav Ther 31(3):441–461, 2000

Nauta H, Hospers H, Jansen A: One-year follow-up effects of two obesity treatments on psychological well-being and weight. Br J Health Psychol 6(Pt 3):271–284, 2001 14596727

Naveed A, Dang N, Gonzalez P, et al: E-cigarette dependence and weight-related attitudes/behaviors associated with eating disorders in adolescent girls. Front Psychiatry 12:713094, 2021 34526923

Nazar BP, Bernardes C, Peachey G, et al: The risk of eating disorders comorbid with attention-deficit/hyper-activity disorder: a systematic review and meta-analysis. Int J Eat Disord 49(12):1045–1057, 2016 27859581

Neiderman M, Zarody M, Tattersall M, et al: Enteric feeding in severe adolescent anorexia nervosa: a report of four cases. Int J Eat Disord 28(4):470–475, 2000 11054797

Neumayr C, Voderholzer U, Tregarthen J, et al: Improving aftercare with technology for anorexia nervosa after intensive inpatient treatment: a pilot randomized controlled trial with a therapist-guided smartphone app. Int J Eat Disord 52(10):1191–1201, 2019 31429974

Nevonen L, Broberg AG: A comparison of sequenced individual and group psychotherapy for patients with bulimia nervosa. Int J Eat Disord 39(2):117–127, 2006 16231341

Nickel C, Tritt K, Muehlbacher M, et al: Topiramate treatment in bulimia nervosa patients: a randomized, double-blind, placebo-controlled trial. Int J Eat Disord 38(4):295–300, 2005 16231337

Nielsen S, Vilmar JW: What can we learn about eating disorder mortality from eating disorder diagnoses at initial assessment? A Danish nationwide register follow-up study using record linkage, encompassing 45 years (1970–2014). Psychiatry Res 303:114091, 2021 34246009

Nikniaz Z, Beheshti S, Abbasalizad Farhangi M, et al: A systematic review and meta-analysis of the prevalence and odds of eating disorders in patients with celiac disease and vice-versa. Int J Eat Disord 54(9):1563–1574, 2021 34042201

Norris ML, Robinson A, Obeid N, et al: Exploring avoidant/restrictive food intake disorder in eating disordered patients: a descriptive study. Int J Eat Disord 47(5):495–499, 2014 24343807

Norris ML, Harrison ME, Isserlin L, et al: Gastrointestinal complications associated with anorexia nervosa: a systematic review. Int J Eat Disord 49(3):216–237, 2016 26407541

Norris ML, Spettigue W, Hammond NG, et al: Building evidence for the use of descriptive subtypes in youth with avoidant restrictive food intake disorder. Int J Eat Disord 51(2):170–173, 2018 29215749

Norris ML, Obeid N, Santos A, et al: Treatment needs and rates of mental health comorbidity in adolescent patients with ARFID. Front Psychiatry 12:680298, 2021 34349680

Nourredine M, Jurek L, Auffret M, et al: Efficacy and safety of topiramate in binge eating disorder: a systematic review and meta-analysis. CNS Spectr 26(5):459–467, 2021 32641176

Nowaskie DZ, Filipowicz AT, Choi Y, et al: Eating disorder symptomatology in transgender patients: differences across gender identity and gender affirmation. Int J Eat Disord 54(8):1493–1499, 2021 33990998

Nyman-Carlsson E, Norring C, Engström I, et al: Individual cognitive behavioral therapy and combined family/individual therapy for young adults with anorexia nervosa: a randomized controlled trial. Psychother Res 30(8):1011–1025, 2020 31709920

Obarzanek E, Lesem MD, Jimerson DC: Resting metabolic rate of anorexia nervosa patients during weight gain. Am J Clin Nutr 60(5):666–675, 1994 7942571

Obeid N, McVey G, Seale E, et al: Cocreating research priorities for anorexia nervosa: the Canadian Eating Disorder Priority Setting Partnership. Int J Eat Disord 53(5):392–402, 2020 32011022

O'Connor G, Nicholls D, Hudson L, et al: Refeeding low weight hospitalized adolescents with anorexia nervosa: a multicenter randomized controlled trial. Nutr Clin Pract 31(5):681–689, 2016 26869609

O'Connor C, McNamara N, O'Hara L, et al: How do people with eating disorders experience the stigma associated with their condition? A mixed-methods systematic review. J Ment Health 30(4):454–469, 2021 31711324

OHSU Center for Diversity and Inclusion: Inclusive language guide. Oregon Health and Science University, February 2021. Available at: https://www.ohsu.edu/inclusive-language-guide. Accessed January 10, 2022.

Olguin P, Fuentes M, Gabler G, et al: Medical comorbidity of binge eating disorder. Eat Weight Disord 22(1):13–26, 2017 27553016

Olivares JL, Vázquez M, Fleta J, et al: Cardiac findings in adolescents with anorexia nervosa at diagnosis and after weight restoration. Eur J Pediatr 164(6):383–386, 2005 15909184

Oliveira SB: Why is avoidant-restrictive food intake disorder relevant to the pediatric gastroenterologist? JAMA Pediatr 175(5):455–457, 2021 33492367

O'Reardon JP, Allison KC, Martino NS, et al: A randomized, placebo-controlled trial of sertraline in the treatment of night eating syndrome. Am J Psychiatry 163(5):893–898, 2006 16648332

O'Reardon JP, Groff KE, Stunkard AJ, et al: Night eating syndrome and results from the first placebo-controlled trial of treatment, with the SSRI medication, sertraline: implications for clinical practice. Progress in Neurotherapeutics and Neuropsychopharmacology 3(1):241–257, 2008

Otsu M, Hamura A, Ishikawa Y, et al: Factors affecting the dental erosion severity of patients with eating disorders. Biopsychosoc Med 8:25, 2014 25904974

Otto AK, Jary JM, Sturza J, et al: Medical admissions among adolescents with eating disorders during the COVID-19 pandemic. Pediatrics 148(4):e2021052201, 2021 34244452

Ozier AD, Henry BW, American Dietetic Association: Position of the American Dietetic Association: nutrition intervention in the treatment of eating disorders. J Am Diet Assoc 111(8):1236–1241, 2011 21802573

Pacilio RM, Livingston RK, Gordon MR: The use of electroconvulsive therapy in eating disorders: a systematic literature review and case report. J ECT 35(4):272–278, 2019 31764451

Padín PF, González-Rodríguez R, Verde-Diego C, et al: Social media and eating disorder psychopathology: a systematic review. Cyberpsychology (Brno) 15(3), 2021

Page MJ, McKenzie JE, Bossuyt PM, et al: The PRISMA 2020 statement: an updated guideline for reporting systematic reviews. BMJ 372(71):n71, 2021 33782057

Painot D, Jotterand S, Kammer A, et al: Simultaneous nutritional cognitive-behavioural therapy in obese patients. Patient Educ Couns 42(1):47–52, 2001 11080605

Patel MM, Brown JD, Croake S, et al: The current state of behavioral health quality measures: where are the gaps? Psychiatr Serv 66(8):865–871, 2015 26073415

Pearlstein T, Spurell E, Hohlstein LA, et al: A double-blind, placebo-controlled trial of fluvoxamine in binge eating disorder: a high placebo response. Arch Women Ment Health 6(2):147–151, 2003 12720065

Peebles R, Sieke EH: Medical complications of eating disorders in youth. Child Adolesc Psychiatr Clin N Am 28(4):593–615, 2019 31443878

Peebles R, Hardy KK, Wilson JL, et al: Are diagnostic criteria for eating disorders markers of medical severity? Pediatrics 125(5):e1193–e1201, 2010 20385643

Peláez-Fernández MA, Javier Labrador F, Raich RM: Validation of eating disorder examination questionnaire (EDE-Q)—Spanish version—for screening eating disorders. Span J Psychol 15(2):817–824, 2012 22774455

Pendleton VR, Goodrick GK, Poston WS, et al: Exercise augments the effects of cognitive-behavioral therapy in the treatment of binge eating. Int J Eat Disord 31(2):172–184, 2002 11920978

Perez M, Ohrt TK, Hoek HW: Prevalence and treatment of eating disorders among Hispanics/Latino Americans in the United States. Curr Opin Psychiatry 29(6):378–382, 2016 27648780

Perry L, Morgan J, Reid F, et al: Screening for symptoms of eating disorders: reliability of the SCOFF screening tool with written compared to oral delivery. Int J Eat Disord 32(4):466–472, 2002 12386911

Pesola GR, Avasarala J: Bupropion seizure proportion among new-onset generalized seizures and drug related seizures presenting to an emergency department. J Emerg Med 22(3):235–239, 2002 11932084

Peters JE, Basnayake C, Hebbard GS, et al: Prevalence of disordered eating in adults with gastrointestinal disorders: a systematic review. Neurogastroenterol Motil 34(8):314278, 2022

Peters K, Meule A, Voderholzer U, et al: Effects of interval-based inpatient treatment for anorexia nervosa: an observational study. Brain Behav 11(11):e2362, 2021 34543514

Peterson CB, Mitchell JE, Engbloom S, et al: Group cognitive-behavioral treatment of binge eating disorder: a comparison of therapist-led versus self-help formats. Int J Eat Disord 24(2):125–136, 1998 9697011

Peterson CB, Mitchell JE, Engbloom S, et al: Self-help versus therapist-led group cognitive-behavioral treatment of binge eating disorder at follow-up. Int J Eat Disord 30(4):363–374, 2001 11746298

Peterson CB, Mitchell JE, Crow SJ, et al: The efficacy of self-help group treatment and therapist-led group treatment for binge eating disorder. Am J Psychiatry 166(12):1347–1354, 2009 19884223

Peterson CB, Engel SG, Crosby RD, et al: Comparing integrative cognitive-affective therapy and guided self-help cognitive-behavioral therapy to treat binge-eating disorder using standard and naturalistic momentary outcome measures: a randomized controlled trial. Int J Eat Disord 53(9):1418–1427, 2020 32583478

Pignatelli AM, Wampers M, Loriedo C, et al: Childhood neglect in eating disorders: a systematic review and meta-analysis. J Trauma Dissociation 18(1):100–115, 2017 27282982

Pike KM, Walsh BT, Vitousek K, et al: Cognitive behavior therapy in the posthospitalization treatment of anorexia nervosa. Am J Psychiatry 160(11):2046–2049, 2003 14594754

Pincus HA, Scholle SH, Spaeth-Rublee B, et al: Quality measures for mental health and substance use: gaps, opportunities, and challenges. Health Aff (Millwood) 35(6):1000–1008, 2016 27269015

Pirotta S, Barillaro M, Brennan L, et al: Disordered eating behaviours and eating disorders in women in Australia with and without polycystic ovary syndrome: a cross-sectional study. J Clin Med 8(10):1682, 2019 31615157

Plummer M: JAGS: Just Another Gibbs Sampler. JAGS, 2021. Available at: https://mcmc-jags.sourceforge.io. Accessed September 26, 2021.

Poulsen S, Lunn S, Daniel SI, et al: A randomized controlled trial of psychoanalytic psychotherapy or cognitive-behavioral therapy for bulimia nervosa. Am J Psychiatry 171(1):109–116, 2014 24275909

Pyle RL, Mitchell JE, Eckert ED, et al: Maintenance treatment and 6-month outcome for bulimic patients who respond to initial treatment. Am J Psychiatry 147(7):871–875, 1990 2192562

Quadflieg N, Strobel C, Naab S, et al: Mortality in males treated for an eating disorder: a large prospective study. Int J Eat Disord 52(12):1365–1369, 2019 31291032

Quesnel D, Cooper M, Dobinson A: Safe exercise at every stage: athlete (SEES-A): a guideline for managing exercise and return to sport in athletes with eating disorders. Safe Exercise at Every Stage, 2019. Available at: https://static1.squarespace.com/static/5b6112bd365f028c9256b26d/t/5f17c005fd8f9a4a19f7d528/1595392150836/Safe+exercise+at+every+stage+-+Athlete.pdf. Accessed January 17, 2022.

Quilty LC, Allen TA, Davis C, et al: A randomized comparison of long acting methylphenidate and cognitive behavioral therapy in the treatment of binge eating disorder. Psychiatry Res 273:467–474, 2019 30684794

Raj KS, Keane-Miller C, Golden NH: Hypomagnesemia in adolescents with eating disorders hospitalized for medical instability. Nutr Clin Pract 27(5):689–694, 2012 22683565

Raj SR, Guzman JC, Harvey P, et al: Canadian Cardiovascular Society position statement on postural orthostatic tachycardia syndrome (POTS) and related disorders of chronic orthostatic intolerance. Can J Cardiol 36(3):357–372, 2020 32145864

Rastogi R, Sieke EH, Nahra A, et al: Return of menses in previously overweight patients with eating disorders. J Pediatr Adolesc Gynecol 33(2):133–138, 2020 31715368

Raykos B, Erceg-Hurn D, McEvoy P, et al: Evidence that the Clinical Impairment Assessment (CIA) subscales should not be scored: bifactor modelling, reliability, and validity in clinical and community samples. Assessment 26(7):1260–1269, 2019 28952332

Raykos BC, Erceg-Hurn DM, Hill J, et al: Positive outcomes from integrating telehealth into routine clinical practice for eating disorders during COVID-19. Int J Eat Disord 54(9):1689–1695, 2021 34184797

R Core Team: R: A Language and Environment for Statistical Computing. Vienna, Austria, R Foundation for Statistical Computing, 2020. Available at: https://www.R-project.org. Accessed September 26, 2021.

Redgrave GW, Coughlin JW, Schreyer CC, et al: Refeeding and weight restoration outcomes in anorexia nervosa: challenging current guidelines. Int J Eat Disord 48(7):866–873, 2015 25625572

Redgrave GW, Schreyer CC, Coughlin JW, et al: Discharge body mass index, not illness chronicity, predicts 6-month weight outcome in patients hospitalized with anorexia nervosa. Front Psychiatry 12:641861, 2021 33716836

Reeves RS, McPherson RS, Nichaman MZ, et al: Nutrient intake of obese female binge eaters. J Am Diet Assoc 101(2):209–215, 2001 11271694

Resmark G, Herpertz S, Herpertz-Dahlmann B, et al: Treatment of anorexia nervosa: new evidence-based guidelines. J Clin Med 8(2):153, 2019 30700054

Ricca V, Mannucci E, Mezzani B, et al: Fluoxetine and fluvoxamine combined with individual cognitive-behaviour therapy in binge eating disorder: a one-year follow-up study. Psychother Psychosom 70(6):298–306, 2001 11598429

Ricca V, Castellini G, Lo Sauro C, et al: Zonisamide combined with cognitive behavioral therapy in binge eating disorder: a one-year follow-up study. Psychiatry (Edgmont) 6(11):23–28, 2009 20049147

Ricca V, Castellini G, Mannucci E, et al: Comparison of individual and group cognitive behavioral therapy for binge eating disorder: a randomized, three-year follow-up study. Appetite 55(3):656–665, 2010 20870000

Ricciardelli LA, McCabe MP, Williams RJ, et al: The role of ethnicity and culture in body image and disordered eating among males. Clin Psychol Rev 27(5):582–606, 2007 17341436

Richards IL, Subar A, Touyz S, et al: Augmentative approaches in family based treatment for adolescents with restrictive eating disorders: a systematic review. Eur Eat Disord Rev 26(2):92–111, 2018 29282801

Richson BN, Johnson SN, Swanson TJ, et al: Predicting probable eating disorder case-status in men using the Clinical Impairment Assessment: evidence for a gender-specific threshold. Eat Behav 42:101541, 2021 34332312

Richter F, Strauss B, Braehler E, et al: Screening disordered eating in a representative sample of the German population: usefulness and psychometric properties of the German SCOFF questionnaire. Eat Behav 25:81–88, 2017 27354266

Riedlinger C, Schmidt G, Weiland A, et al: Which symptoms, complaints and complications of the gastrointestinal tract occur in patients with eating disorders? A systematic review and quantitative analysis. Front Psychiatry 11:195, 2020 32425816

Rigaud D, Brondel L, Poupard AT, et al: A randomized trial on the efficacy of a 2-month tube feeding regimen in anorexia nervosa: a 1-year follow-up study. Clin Nutr 26(4):421–429, 2007a 17499892

Rigaud D, Verges B, Colas-Linhart N, et al: Hormonal and psychological factors linked to the increased thermic effect of food in malnourished fasting anorexia nervosa. J Clin Endocrinol Metab 92(5):1623–1629, 2007b 17341571

Rio A, Whelan K, Goff L, et al: Occurrence of refeeding syndrome in adults started on artificial nutrition support: prospective cohort study. BMJ Open 3(1):e002173, 2013 23315514

Riquin E, Raynal A, Mattar L, et al: Is the severity of the clinical expression of anorexia nervosa influenced by an anxiety, depressive, or obsessive-compulsive comorbidity over a lifetime? Front Psychiatry 12:658416, 2021 34279519

Robb AS, Silber TJ, Orrell-Valente JK, et al: Supplemental nocturnal nasogastric refeeding for better short-term outcome in hospitalized adolescent girls with anorexia nervosa. Am J Psychiatry 159(8):1347–1353, 2002 12153827

Robin AL, Siegel PT, Koepke T, et al: Family therapy versus individual therapy for adolescent females with anorexia nervosa. J Dev Behav Pediatr 15(2):111–116, 1994 8034762

Robin AL, Siegel PT, Moye A: Family versus individual therapy for anorexia: impact on family conflict. Int J Eat Disord 17(4):313–322, 1995 7620470

Robin AL, Siegel PT, Moye AW, et al: A controlled comparison of family versus individual therapy for adolescents with anorexia nervosa. J Am Acad Child Adolesc Psychiatry 38(12):1482–1489, 1999 10596247

Robinson L, Aldridge V, Clark EM, et al: A systematic review and meta-analysis of the association between eating disorders and bone density. Osteoporos Int 27(6):1953–1966, 2016 26782684

Robinson L, Aldridge VK, Clark EM, et al: Bone health in adult women with ED: a longitudinal community-based study. J Psychosom Res 116:115–122, 2019 30577982

Robson J, Laborda T, Fitzgerald S, et al: Avoidant/restrictive food intake disorder in diet-treated children with eosinophilic esophagitis. J Pediatr Gastroenterol Nutr 69(1):57–60, 2019 30889128

Romano SJ, Halmi KA, Sarkar NP, et al: A placebo-controlled study of fluoxetine in continued treatment of bulimia nervosa after successful acute fluoxetine treatment. Am J Psychiatry 159(1):96–102, 2002 11772696

Rosen E, Sabel AL, Brinton JT, et al: Liver dysfunction in patients with severe anorexia nervosa. Int J Eat Disord 49(2):151–158, 2016 26346046

Royal Colleges of Psychiatrists: College Report (CR189) on MARSIPAN: Management of Really Sick Patients with Anorexia Nervosa, 2nd Edition. London, Royal College of Psychiatrists, 2014. Available at: https://www.rcpsych.ac.uk/docs/default-source/improving-care/better-mh-policy/college-reports/college-report-cr189.pdf?sfvrsn=6c2e7ada_2. Accessed August 18, 2021.

Ruggiero GM, Laini V, Mauri MC, et al: A single blind comparison of amisulpride, fluoxetine and clomipramine in the treatment of restricting anorectics. Prog Neuropsychopharmacol Biol Psychiatry 25(5):1049–1059, 2001 11444677

Ruggiero GM, Mauri MC, Omboni AC, et al: Nutritional management of anorexic patients with and without fluoxetine: 1-year follow-up. Prog Neuropsychopharmacol Biol Psychiatry 27(3):425–430, 2003 12691777

Russell GF, Szmukler GI, Dare C, et al: An evaluation of family therapy in anorexia nervosa and bulimia nervosa. Arch Gen Psychiatry 44(12):1047–1056, 1987 3318754

Russon J, Mensinger J, Herres J, et al: Identifying risk factors for disordered eating among female youth in primary care. Child Psychiatry Hum Dev 50(5):727–737, 2019 30847634

Sachs K, Mehler PS: Medical complications of bulimia nervosa and their treatments. Eat Weight Disord 21(1):13–18, 2016 26166603

Sachs KV, Harnke B, Mehler PS, et al: Cardiovascular complications of anorexia nervosa: a systematic review. Int J Eat Disord 49(3):238–248, 2016 26710932

Safer DL, Telch CF, Agras WS: Dialectical behavior therapy for bulimia nervosa. Am J Psychiatry 158(4):632–634, 2001 11282700

Safer DL, Robinson AH, Jo B: Outcome from a randomized controlled trial of group therapy for binge eating disorder: comparing dialectical behavior therapy adapted for binge eating to an active comparison group therapy. Behav Ther 41(1):106–120, 2010 20171332

Safer DL, Adler S, Dalai SS, et al: A randomized, placebo-controlled crossover trial of phentermine-topiramate ER in patients with binge-eating disorder and bulimia nervosa. Int J Eat Disord 53(2):266–277, 2020 31721257

Salerno L, Rhind C, Hibbs R, et al: A longitudinal examination of dyadic distress patterns following a skills intervention for carers of adolescents with anorexia nervosa. Eur Child Adolesc Psychiatry 25(12):1337–1347, 2016 27161339

Santomauro DF, Melen S, Mitchison D, et al: The hidden burden of eating disorders: an extension of estimates from the Global Burden of Disease Study 2019. Lancet Psychiatry 8(4):320–328, 2021 33675688

Sawyer SM, Whitelaw M, Le Grange D, et al: Physical and psychological morbidity in adolescents with atypical anorexia nervosa. Pediatrics 137(4):e20154080, 2016 27025958

Schaefer LM, Steinglass JE: Reward learning through the lens of RDoC: a review of theory, assessment, and empirical findings in the eating disorders. Curr Psychiatry Rep 23(1):2, 2021 33386514

Schaefer LM, Smith KE, Leonard R, et al: Identifying a male clinical cutoff on the Eating Disorder Examination-Questionnaire (EDE-Q). Int J Eat Disord 51(12):1357–1360, 2018 30480321

Schaefer LM, Crosby RD, Machado PPP: A systematic review of instruments for the assessment of eating disorders among adults. Curr Opin Psychiatry 34(6):543–562, 2021 34475351

Schag K, Rennhak SK, Leehr EJ, et al: IMPULS: impulsivity-focused group intervention to reduce binge eating episodes in patients with binge eating disorder: a randomised controlled trial. Psychother Psychosom 88(3):141–153, 2019 31108488

Schalla MA, Stengel A: Gastrointestinal alterations in anorexia nervosa: a systematic review. Eur Eat Disord Rev 27(5):447–461, 2019 31062912

Schebendach JE, Golden NH, Jacobson MS, et al: The metabolic responses to starvation and refeeding in adolescents with anorexia nervosa. Ann N Y Acad Sci 817:110–119, 1997 9239182

Schebendach JE, Mayer LE, Devlin MJ, et al: Dietary energy density and diet variety as predictors of outcome in anorexia nervosa. Am J Clin Nutr 87(4):810–816, 2008 18400701 Erratum in Am J Clin Nutr 96(1):222, 2012

Schebendach JE, Mayer LE, Devlin MJ, et al: Food choice and diet variety in weight-restored patients with anorexia nervosa. J Am Diet Assoc 111(5):732–736, 2011 21515121

Schebendach JE, Mayer LE, Devlin MJ, et al: Dietary energy density and diet variety as risk factors for relapse in anorexia nervosa: a replication. Int J Eat Disord 45(1):79–84, 2012 21448937

Schlup B, Munsch S, Meyer AH, et al: The efficacy of a short version of a cognitive-behavioral treatment followed by booster sessions for binge eating disorder. Behav Res Ther 47(7):628–635, 2009 19446793

Schlup B, Meyer AH, Munsch S: A non-randomized direct comparison of cognitive-behavioral short- and long-term treatment for binge eating disorder. Obes Facts 3(4):261–266, 2010 20823690

Schmidt U, Treasure J: Getting Better Bit(e) by Bit(e): A Treatment Manual for Sufferers of Bulimia Nervosa. Hove, East Sussex, UK, Psychology Press, 1997

Schmidt U, Cooper PJ, Essers H, et al: Fluvoxamine and graded psychotherapy in the treatment of bulimia nervosa: a randomized, double-blind, placebo-controlled, multicenter study of short-term and long-term pharmacotherapy combined with a stepped care approach to psychotherapy. J Clin Psychopharmacol 24(5):549–552, 2004 15349014

Schmidt U, Lee S, Beecham J, et al: A randomized controlled trial of family therapy and cognitive behavior therapy guided self-care for adolescents with bulimia nervosa and related disorders. Am J Psychiatry 164(4):591–598, 2007 17403972

Schmidt U, Oldershaw A, Jichi F, et al: Out-patient psychological therapies for adults with anorexia nervosa: randomised controlled trial. Br J Psychiatry 201(5):392–399, 2012 22995632

Schmidt U, Magill N, Renwick B, et al: The Maudsley Outpatient Study of Treatments for Anorexia Nervosa and Related Conditions (MOSAIC): comparison of the Maudsley Model of Anorexia Nervosa Treatment for Adults (MANTRA) with specialist supportive clinical management (SSCM) in outpatients with broadly defined anorexia nervosa: a randomized controlled trial. J Consult Clin Psychol 83(4):796–807, 2015 25984803

Schmidt U, Ryan EG, Bartholdy S, et al: Two-year follow-up of the MOSAIC trial: a multicenter randomized controlled trial comparing two psychological treatments in adult outpatients with broadly defined anorexia nervosa. Int J Eat Disord 49(8):793–800, 2016 27061709

Schmidt R, Hiemisch A, Kiess W, et al: Macro- and micronutrient intake in children with avoidant/restrictive food intake disorder. Nutrients 13(2):400, 2021 33513954

Schneider W, Klauer T, Freyberger HJ: Operationalized psychodynamic diagnosis in planning and evaluating the psychotherapeutic process. Eur Arch Psychiatry Clin Neurosci 258(Suppl 5):86–91, 2008 18985302

Schorr M, Miller KK: The endocrine manifestations of anorexia nervosa: mechanisms and management. Nat Rev Endocrinol 13(3):174–186, 2017 27811940

Scott CL, Haycraft E, Plateau CR: Teammate influences and relationship quality are associated with eating and exercise psychopathology in athletes. Appetite 143:104404, 2019 31421196

Sharp WG, Stubbs KH, Adams H, et al: Intensive, manual-based intervention for pediatric feeding disorders: results from a randomized pilot trial. J Pediatr Gastroenterol Nutr 62(4):658–663, 2016 26628445

Shilton T, Enoch-Levy A, Giron Y, et al: A retrospective case series of electroconvulsive therapy in the management of comorbid depression and anorexia nervosa. Int J Eat Disord 53(2):210–218, 2020 31639233

Shim KS: Pubertal growth and epiphyseal fusion. Ann Pediatr Endocrinol Metab 20(1):8–12, 2015 25883921

Shimshoni Y, Lebowitz ER: Childhood avoidant/restrictive food intake disorder: review of treatments and a novel parent-based approach. J Cogn Psychother 34(3):200–224, 2020 32817402

Shimshoni Y, Silverman WK, Lebowitz ER: SPACE-ARFID: a pilot trial of a novel parent-based treatment for avoidant/restrictive food intake disorder. Int J Eat Disord 53(10):1623–1635, 2020 33464594

Singer W, Sletten DM, Opfer-Gehrking TL, et al: Postural tachycardia in children and adolescents: what is abnormal? J Pediatr 160(2):222–226, 2012 21996154

Singhal V, Bose A, Slattery M, et al: Effect of transdermal estradiol and insulin-like growth factor-1 on bone endpoints of young women with anorexia nervosa. J Clin Endocrinol Metab 106(7):2021–2035, 2021 33693703

Smith AR, Zuromski KL, Dodd DR: Eating disorders and suicidality: what we know, what we don't know, and suggestions for future research. Curr Opin Psychol 22:63–67, 2018 28846874

Smith KE, Mason TB, Murray SB, et al: Male clinical norms and sex differences on the Eating Disorder Inventory (EDI) and Eating Disorder Examination Questionnaire (EDE-Q). Int J Eat Disord 50(7):769–775, 2017 28436086

Smythe J, Colebourn C, Prisco L, et al: Cardiac abnormalities identified with echocardiography in anorexia nervosa: systematic review and meta-analysis. Br J Psychiatry 219(3):477–486, 2021 32026793

Society for Adolescent Health and Medicine: Refeeding hypophosphatemia in hospitalized adolescents with anorexia nervosa: a position statement of the Society for Adolescent Health and Medicine. J Adolesc Health 55(3):455–457, 2014 25151056

Solmi F, Hatch SL, Hotopf M, et al: Validation of the SCOFF questionnaire for eating disorders in a multiethnic general population sample. Int J Eat Disord 48(3):312–316, 2015 25504212

Solmi M, Veronese N, Correll CU, et al: Bone mineral density, osteoporosis, and fractures among people with eating disorders: a systematic review and meta-analysis. Acta Psychiatr Scand 133(5):341–351, 2016 26763350

Solmi M, Radua J, Stubbs B, et al: Risk factors for eating disorders: an umbrella review of published meta-analyses. Br J Psychiatry 43(3):314–323, 2021 32997075

Spettigue W, Norris ML, Santos A, et al: Treatment of children and adolescents with avoidant/restrictive food intake disorder: a case series examining the feasibility of family therapy and adjunctive treatments. J Eat Disord 6:20, 2018 30123505

Spettigue W, Norris ML, Douziech I, et al: Feasibility of implementing a family based inpatient program for adolescents with anorexia nervosa: a retrospective cohort study. Front Psychiatry 10:887, 2019 31849732

Stefini A, Salzer S, Reich G, et al: Cognitive-behavioral and psychodynamic therapy in female adolescents with bulimia nervosa: a randomized controlled trial. J Am Acad Child Adolesc Psychiatry 56(4):329–335, 2017 28335877

Steinglass JE, Kaplan SC, Liu Y, et al: The (lack of) effect of alprazolam on eating behavior in anorexia nervosa: a preliminary report. Int J Eat Disord 47(8):901–904, 2014 25139178

Steinhausen HC, Villumsen MD, Hørder K, et al: Comorbid mental disorders during long-term course in a nationwide cohort of patients with anorexia nervosa. Int J Eat Disord 54(9):1608–1618, 2021 34145619

Sterne JAC, Savovic J, Page MJ, et al: RoB 2: a revised tool for assessing risk of bias in randomised trials. BMJ 366:l4898, 2019 31462531

Stewart C, Konstantellou A, Kassamali F, et al: Is this the "new normal"? A mixed method investigation of young person, parent and clinician experience of online eating disorder treatment during the COVID-19 pandemic. J Eat Disord 9(1):78, 2021 34193291

Stice E, Onipede ZA, Marti CN: A meta-analytic review of trials that tested whether eating disorder prevention programs prevent eating disorder onset. Clin Psychol Rev 87:102046, 2021 34048952

Stiles-Shields C, Touyz S, Hay P, et al: Therapeutic alliance in two treatments for adults with severe and enduring anorexia nervosa. Int J Eat Disord 46(8):783–789, 2013 24014042

Strandjord SE, Sieke EH, Richmond M, Rome ES: Avoidant/restrictive food intake disorder: illness and hospital course in patients hospitalized for nutritional insufficiency. J Adolesc Health 57(6):673–678, 2015 26422290

Strandjord SE, Sieke EH, Richmond M, et al: Medical stabilization of adolescents with nutritional insufficiency: a clinical care path. Eat Weight Disord 21(3):403–410, 2016 26597679

Streatfeild J, Hickson J, Austin SB, et al: Social and economic cost of eating disorders in the United States: evidence to inform policy action. Int J Eat Disord 54(5):851–868, 2021 33655603

Strokosch GR, Friedman AJ, Wu SC, Kamin M: Effects of an oral contraceptive (norgestimate/ethinyl estradiol) on bone mineral density in adolescent females with anorexia nervosa: a double-blind, placebo-controlled study. J Adolesc Health 39(6):819–827, 2006 17116511

Sundgot-Borgen J, Torstveit MK: Prevalence of eating disorders in elite athletes is higher than in the general population. Clin J Sport Med 14(1):25–32, 2004 14712163

Sundgot-Borgen J, Rosenvinge JH, Bahr R, et al: The effect of exercise, cognitive therapy, and nutritional counseling in treating bulimia nervosa. Med Sci Sports Exerc 34(2):190–195, 2002 11828224

Suter PM, Russell RM: Vitamin and trace mineral deficiency and excess, in Harrison's Principles of Internal Medicine, 20th Edition. Edited by Jameson J, Fauci AS, Kasper DL, et al. New York, McGraw-Hill, 2018. Available at: https://accessmedicine.mhmedical.com/content.aspx?bookid=1130&sectionid=63653455. Accessed February 27, 2021.

Swenne I, Thurfjell B: Clinical onset and diagnosis of eating disorders in premenarcheal girls is preceded by inadequate weight gain and growth retardation. Acta Paediatr 92(10):1133–1137, 2003 14632326

Sysko R, Glasofer DR, Hildebrandt T, et al: The eating disorder assessment for DSM-5 (EDA-5): development and validation of a structured interview for feeding and eating disorders. Int J Eat Disord 48(5):452–463, 2015 25639562

Szmukler GI, Young GP, Miller G, et al: A controlled trial of cisapride in anorexia nervosa. Int J Eat Disord 17(4):347–357, 1995 7620474

Takeda Pharmaceuticals: Vyvanse (lisdexamfetamine) prescribing information. Lexington, MA, Takeda Pharmaceutials America Inc, July 2021. Available at: https://www.accessdata.fda.gov/drugsatfda_docs/label/2021/021977s046,208510s003lbl.pdf.

Tannous WK, Hay P, Girosi F, et al: The economic cost of bulimia nervosa and binge eating disorder: a population-based study. Psychol Med May 17, 2021 33998425

Taquet M, Geddes JR, Luciano S, et al: Incidence and outcomes of eating disorders during the COVID-19 pandemic. Br J Psychiatry 200(5):1–3, 2021 7620474

Tasca GA, Ritchie K, Conrad G, et al: Attachment scales predict outcome in a randomized controlled trial of two group therapies for binge eating disorder: an aptitude by treatment interaction. Psychother Res 16(1):106–121, 2006

Tasca GA, Balfour L, Presniak MD, et al: Outcomes of specific interpersonal problems for binge eating disorder: comparing group psychodynamic interpersonal psychotherapy and group cognitive behavioral therapy. Int J Group Psychother 62(2):197–218, 2012 22468572

Tasca GA, Koszycki D, Brugnera A, et al: Testing a stepped care model for binge-eating disorder: a two-step randomized controlled trial. Psychol Med 49(4):598–606, 2019 29792242

Tatham M, Turner H, Mountford VA, et al: Development, psychometric properties and preliminary clinical validation of a brief, session-by-session measure of eating disorder cognitions and behaviors: the ED-15. Int J Eat Disord 48(7):1005–1015, 2015 26011054

Taylor JY, Caldwell CH, Baser RE, et al: Prevalence of eating disorders among Blacks in the National Survey of American Life. Int J Eat Disord 40(Suppl):S10–S14, 2007 17879287

Telch CF, Agras WS, Rossiter EM, et al: Group cognitive-behavioral treatment for the nonpurging bulimic: an initial evaluation. J Consult Clin Psychol 58(5):629–635, 1990 2254511

Telch CF, Agras WS, Linehan MM: Dialectical behavior therapy for binge eating disorder. J Consult Clin Psychol 69(6):1061–1065, 2001 11777110

Thackwray DE, Smith MC, Bodfish JW, et al: A comparison of behavioral and cognitive-behavioral interventions for bulimia nervosa. J Consult Clin Psychol 61(4):639–645, 1993 8370859

Thannickal A, Brutocao C, Alsawas M, et al: Eating, sleeping and sexual function disorders in women with polycystic ovary syndrome (PCOS): a systematic review and meta-analysis. Clin Endocrinol (Oxf) 92(4):338–349, 2020 31917860

Thiels C, Schmidt U, Treasure J, et al: Guided self-change for bulimia nervosa incorporating use of a self-care manual. Am J Psychiatry 155(7):947–953, 1998 9659862

Thiels C, Schmidt U, Troop N, et al: Binge frequency predicts outcome in guided self-care treatment of bulimia nervosa. Eur Eat Disord Rev 8(4):272–278, 2000

Thiels C, Schmidt U, Treasure J, et al: Four-year follow-up of guided self-change for bulimia nervosa. Eat Weight Disord 8(3):212–217, 2003 14649785

Thomas JJ, Becker KR, Kuhnle MC, et al: Cognitive-behavioral therapy for avoidant/restrictive food intake disorder: feasibility, acceptability, and proof-of-concept for children and adolescents. Int J Eat Disord 53(10):1636–1646, 2020 32776570

Thomas JJ, Becker KR, Breithaupt L, et al: Cognitive-behavioral therapy for adults with avoidant/restrictive food intake disorder. J Behav Cogn Ther 31(1):47–55, 2021 34423319

Thompson-Brenner H, Shingleton RM, Thompson DR, et al: Focused vs. broad enhanced cognitive behavioral therapy for bulimia nervosa with comorbid borderline personality: a randomized controlled trial. Int J Eat Disord 49(1):36–49, 2016 26649812

Tinsley GM, Smith-Ryan AE, Kim Y, et al: Fat-free mass characteristics vary based on sex, race, and weight status in US adults. Nutr Res 81:58–70, 2020 32882467

Tith RM, Paradis G, Potter BJ, et al: Association of bulimia nervosa with long-term risk of cardiovascular disease and mortality among women. JAMA Psychiatry 77(1):44–51, 2020 31617882

Toni G, Berioli MG, Cerquiglini L, et al: Eating disorders and disordered eating symptoms in adolescents with Type 1 diabetes. Nutrients 9(8):906, 2017 28825608

Toulany A, Kurdyak P, Guttmann A, et al: Acute care visits for eating disorders among children and adolescents after the onset of the COVID-19 pandemic. J Adolesc Health 70(1):42–47, 2022 34690054

Touyz S, Le Grange D, Lacey H, et al: Treating severe and enduring anorexia nervosa: a randomized controlled trial. Psychol Med 43(12):2501–2511, 2013 23642330

Traboulsi S, Itani L, Tannir H, et al: Is body fat percentage a good predictor of menstrual recovery in females with anorexia nervosa after weight restoration? A systematic review and exploratory and selective meta-analysis. J Popul Ther Clin Pharmacol 26(2):e25–e37, 2019 31577083

Treasure J, Schmidt U, Troop N, et al: First step in managing bulimia nervosa: controlled trial of therapeutic manual. BMJ 308(6930):686–689, 1994 8142791

Treasure J, Todd G, Brolly M, et al: A pilot study of a randomised trial of cognitive analytical therapy vs educational behavioral therapy for adult anorexia nervosa. Behav Res Ther 33(4):363–367, 1995 7755523

Treasure J, Smith G, Crane A: Skills-Based Learning for Caring for a Loved One With an Eating Disorder: The New Maudsley Method. New York, Routledge, 2007

Udo T, Grilo CM: Prevalence and correlates of DSM-5-defined eating disorders in a nationally representative sample of U.S. adults. Biol Psychiatry 84(5):345–354, 2018 29859631

Udo T, Grilo CM: Psychiatric and medical correlates of DSM-5 eating disorders in a nationally representative sample of adults in the United States. Int J Eat Disord 52(1):42–50, 2019 30756422

Udo T, Bitley S, Grilo CM: Suicide attempts in US adults with lifetime DSM-5 eating disorders. BMC Med 17(1):120, 2019 31234891

Uniacke B, Glasofer D, Devlin M, et al: Predictors of eating-related psychopathology in transgender and gender nonbinary individuals. Eat Behav 42:101527, 2021 34049054

U.S. Food and Drug Administration: Suicidality in children and adolescents being treated with antidepressant medications. U.S. Food and Drug Administration, February 2018. Available at: https://www.fda.gov/drugs/postmarket-drug-safety-information-patients-and-providers/suicidality-children-and-adolescents-being-treated-antidepressant-medications. Accessed August 15, 2021.

U.S. Preventive Services Task Force: Eating Disorders in Adolescents and Adults: Screening. Rockville, MD, U.S. Preventive Services Task Force, 2022

van Dulmen SA, Lukersmith S, Muxlow J, et al: Supporting a person-centred approach in clinical guidelines: a position paper of the Allied Health Community Guidelines International Network (G-I-N). Health Expect 18(5):1543–1558, 2015 24118821

van Furth EF, van der Meer A, Cowan K: Top 10 research priorities for eating disorders. Lancet Psychiatry 3(8):706–707, 2016 27475763

van Hoeken D, Hoek HW: Review of the burden of eating disorders: mortality, disability, costs, quality of life, and family burden. Curr Opin Psychiatry 33(6):521–527, 2020 32796186

Van Wymelbeke V, Brondel L, Marcel Brun J, et al: Factors associated with the increase in resting energy expenditure during refeeding in malnourished anorexia nervosa patients. Am J Clin Nutr 80(6):1469–1477, 2004 15585757

Vander Wal JS, Gang CH, Griffing GT, et al: Escitalopram for treatment of night eating syndrome: a 12-week, randomized, placebo-controlled trial. J Clin Psychopharmacol 32(3):341–345, 2012 22544016

Vestergaard P, Emborg C, Støving RK, et al: Patients with eating disorders: a high-risk group for fractures. Orthop Nurs 22(5):325–331, 2003 14595992

Volkert VM, Burrell L, Berry RC, et al: Intensive multidisciplinary feeding intervention for patients with avoidant/restrictive food intake disorder associated with severe food selectivity: an electronic health record review. Int J Eat Disord 54(11):1978–1988, 2021 34505302

Wadden TA, Faulconbridge LF, Jones-Corneille LR, et al: Binge eating disorder and the outcome of bariatric surgery at one year: a prospective, observational study. Obesity (Silver Spring) 19(6):1220–1228, 2011 21253005

Wade TD, Allen K, Crosby RD, et al: Outpatient therapy for adult anorexia nervosa: early weight gain trajectories and outcome. Eur Eat Disord Rev 29(3):472–481, 2021 32838476

Wagner G, Penelo E, Wanner C, et al: Internet-delivered cognitive-behavioural therapy v. conventional guided self-help for bulimia nervosa: long-term evaluation of a randomised controlled trial. Br J Psychiatry 202:135–141, 2013 23222037

Wagner B, Nagl M, Dölemeyer R, et al: Randomized controlled trial of an internet-based cognitive-behavioral treatment program for binge-eating disorder. Behav Ther 47(4):500–514, 2016 27423166

Wagner AF, Lane-Loney SE, Essayli JH: Patient perceptions of blind and open weighing in treatment for eating disorders. Eat Disord 30(2):230–238, 2022 34702149

Walker DC, Heiss S, Donahue JM, et al: Practitioners' perspectives on ethical issues within the treatment of eating disorders: results from a concept mapping study. Int J Eat Disord 53(12):1941–1951, 2020 32918314

Waller G, Pugh M, Mulkens S, et al: Cognitive-behavioral therapy in the time of coronavirus: clinician tips for working with eating disorders via telehealth when face-to-face meetings are not possible. Int J Eat Disord 53(7):1132–1141, 2020 32383530

Wallin U, Holmer R: Long-term outcome of adolescent anorexia nervosa: family treatment apartments compared with child psychiatric inpatient treatment. Front Psychiatry 12:640622, 2021 34079480

Wallin U, Kronovall P, Majewski ML: Body awareness therapy in teenage anorexia nervosa: outcome after 2 years. Eur Eat Disord Rev 8(1):19–30, 2000

Walsh BT, Stewart JW, Roose SP, et al: Treatment of bulimia with phenelzine: a double-blind, placebo-controlled study. Arch Gen Psychiatry 41(11):1105–1109, 1984 6388524

Walsh BT, Stewart JW, Roose SP, et al: A double-blind trial of phenelzine in bulimia. J Psychiatr Res 19(2–3):485–489, 1985 3900362

Walsh BT, Gladis M, Roose SP, et al: Phenelzine vs placebo in 50 patients with bulimia. Arch Gen Psychiatry 45(5):471–475, 1988 3282482

Walsh BT, Wilson GT, Loeb KL, et al: Medication and psychotherapy in the treatment of bulimia nervosa. Am J Psychiatry 154(4):523–531, 1997 9090340

Walsh BT, Agras WS, Devlin MJ, et al: Fluoxetine for bulimia nervosa following poor response to psychotherapy. Am J Psychiatry 157(8):1332–1334, 2000 10910801

Walsh BT, Kaplan Allan S, Attia E, et al: Fluoxetine after weight restoration in anorexia nervosa: a randomized controlled trial.JAMA 295(22):2605–2612, 2006 16772623. Erratum in JAMA 296(8):934, 2006

Wang Z, Whiteside SPH, Sim L, et al: Comparative effectiveness and safety of cognitive behavioral therapy and pharmacotherapy for childhood anxiety disorders: a systematic review and meta-analysis. JAMA Pediatr 17111:1049–1056, 2017 28859190. Erratum in JAMA Pediatr 17210:992, 2018

Ward A, Ramsay R, Russell G, et al: Follow-up mortality study of compulsorily treated patients with anorexia nervosa. Int J Eat Disord 48(7):860–865, 2015 25545619

Ward ZJ, Rodriguez P, Wright DR, et al: Estimation of eating disorders prevalence by age and associations with mortality in a simulated nationally representative US cohort. JAMA Netw Open 2(10):e1912925, 2019 31596495

Wasil AR, Patel R, Cho JY, et al: Smartphone apps for eating disorders: a systematic review of evidence-based content and application of user-adjusted analyses. Int J Eat Disord 54(5):690–700, 2021 33534176

Watkins K, Horvitz-Lennon M, Caldarone LB, et al: Developing medical record-based performance indicators to measure the quality of mental healthcare. J Healthc Qual 33(1):49–66, quiz 66–67, 2011 21199073

Watkins KE, Farmer CM, De Vries D, et al: The Affordable Care Act: an opportunity for improving care for substance use disorders? Psychiatr Serv 66(3):310–312, 2015 25727120

Watkins KE, Smith B, Akincigil A, et al: The quality of medication treatment for mental disorders in the Department of Veterans Affairs and in private-sector plans. Psychiatr Serv 67(4):391–396, 2016 26567931

Watson HJ, Joyce T, French E, et al: Prevention of eating disorders: a systematic review of randomized, controlled trials. Int J Eat Disord 49(9):833–862, 2016 27425572

Watson HJ, Levine MD, Zerwas SC, et al: Predictors of dropout in face-to-face and internet-based cognitive-behavioral therapy for bulimia nervosa in a randomized controlled trial. Int J Eat Disord 50(5):569–577, 2017 27862108

Waxman SE: A systematic review of impulsivity in eating disorders. Eur Eat Disord Rev 17(6):408–425, 2009 19548249

Weinsier RL, Krumdieck CL: Death resulting from overzealous total parenteral nutrition: the refeeding syndrome revisited. Am J Clin Nutr 34(3):393–399, 1981 6782855

West M, McMaster CM, Staudacher HM, et al: Gastrointestinal symptoms following treatment for anorexia nervosa: a systematic literature review. Int J Eat Disord 54(6):936–951, 2021 33529388

Westmoreland P, Krantz MJ, Mehler PS: Medical complications of anorexia nervosa and bulimia. Am J Med 129(1):30–37, 2016 26169883

White MA, Grilo CM: Bupropion for overweight women with binge-eating disorder: a randomized, double-blind, placebo-controlled trial. J Clin Psychiatry 74(4):400–406, 2013 23656848

Whitelaw M, Gilbertson H, Lee KJ, et al: Restrictive eating disorders among adolescent inpatients. Pediatrics 134(3):e758–e764, 2014 25157005

Whitelaw M, Lee KJ, Gilbertson H, et al: Predictors of complications in anorexia nervosa and atypical anorexia nervosa: degree of underweight or extent and recency of weight loss? J Adolesc Health 63(6):717–723, 2018 30454732

Wild B, Friederich HC, Gross G, et al: The ANTOP study: focal psychodynamic psychotherapy, cognitive-behavioural therapy, and treatment-as-usual in outpatients with anorexia nervosa: a randomized controlled trial. Trials 10:23, 2009 19389245

Wildes JE, Marcus MD: Application of the Research Domain Criteria (RDoC) framework to eating disorders: emerging concepts and research. Curr Psychiatry Rep 17(5):30, 2015 25773226

Wilfley DE, Agras WS, Telch CF, et al: Group cognitive-behavioral therapy and group interpersonal psychotherapy for the nonpurging bulimic individual: a controlled comparison. J Consult Clin Psychol 61(2):296–305, 1993 8473584

Wilfley DE, Welch RR, Stein RI, et al: A randomized comparison of group cognitive-behavioral therapy and group interpersonal psychotherapy for the treatment of overweight individuals with binge-eating disorder. Arch Gen Psychiatry 59(8):713–721, 2002 12150647

Wilson GT, Loeb KL, Walsh BT, et al: Psychological versus pharmacological treatments of bulimia nervosa: predictors and processes of change. J Consult Clin Psychol 67(4):451–459, 1999 10450615

Wilson GT, Fairburn CC, Agras WS, et al: Cognitive-behavioral therapy for bulimia nervosa: time course and mechanisms of change. J Consult Clin Psychol 70(2):267–274, 2002 11952185

Wilson GT, Wilfley DE, Agras WS, et al: Psychological treatments of binge eating disorder. Arch Gen Psychiatry 67(1):94–101, 2010 20048227

Wonderlich SA, Peterson CB, Crosby RD, et al: A randomized controlled comparison of integrative cognitive-affective therapy (ICAT) and enhanced cognitive-behavioral therapy (CBT-E) for bulimia nervosa. Psychol Med 44(3):543–553, 2014 23701891. Erratum in Psychol Med 44(11):2462–2463, 2014

Woosley RL, Heise CW, Gallo T, et al: QTdrugs list. Available at: https://www.crediblemeds.org. Accessed January 8, 2022.

Workman C, Blalock DV, Mehler PS: Bone density status in a large population of patients with anorexia nervosa. Bone 131:115161, 2020 31765843

Wu J, Liu J, Li S, et al: Trends in the prevalence and disability-adjusted life years of eating disorders from 1990 to 2017: results from the Global Burden of Disease Study 2017. Epidemiol Psychiatr Sci 29:e191, 2020 33283690

Wyssen A, Meyer AH, Messerli-Bürgy N, et al: BED-online: acceptance and efficacy of an internet-based treatment for binge-eating disorder: a randomized clinical trial including waitlist conditions. Eur Eat Disord Rev 29(6):937–954, 2021 34418221

Yager J, Devlin MJ, Halmi KA, et al: Guideline Watch (August 2012): Practice Guideline for the Treatment of Patients With Eating Disorders, 3rd Edition. Washington, DC, American Psychiatric Association, 2012

Yelencich E, Truong E, Widaman AM, et al: Avoidant restrictive food intake disorder prevalent among patients with inflammatory bowel disease. Clin Gastroenterol Hepatol 20(6):1282.e1–1289.e1, 2022 34389486

Yoon C, Mason SM, Hooper L, et al: Disordered eating behaviors and 15-year trajectories in body mass index: findings from Project Eating and Activity in Teens and Young Adults (EAT). J Adolesc Health 66(2):181–188, 2020 31630924

Young V, Eiser C, Johnson B, et al: Eating problems in adolescents with Type 1 diabetes: a systematic review with meta-analysis. Diabet Med 30(2):189–198, 2013 22913589

Yu J, Stewart Agras W, Halmi KA, et al: A 1-year follow-up of a multi-center treatment trial of adults with anorexia nervosa. Eat Weight Disord 16(3):e177–e181, 2011 22290033

Yule S, Wanik J, Holm EM, et al: Nutritional deficiency disease secondary to ARFID symptoms associated with autism and the broad autism phenotype: a qualitative systematic review of case reports and case series. J Acad Nutr Diet 121(3):467–492, 2021 33221247

Zeeck A, Weber S, Sandholz A, et al: Inpatient versus day clinic treatment for bulimia nervosa: a randomized trial. Psychother Psychosom 78(3):152–160, 2009a 19270470

Zeeck A, Weber S, Sandholz A, et al: Inpatient versus day treatment for bulimia nervosa: results of a one-year follow-up. Psychother Psychosom 78(5):317–319, 2009b 19628960

Zeeck A, Hartmann A, Wild B, et al: How do patients with anorexia nervosa "process" psychotherapy between sessions? A comparison of cognitive-behavioral and psychodynamic interventions. Psychother Res 28(6):873–886, 2018 27808005

Zerwas SC, Watson HJ, Hofmeier SM, et al: CBT4BN: a randomized controlled trial of online chat and face-to-face group therapy for bulimia nervosa. Psychother Psychosom 86(1):47–53, 2017 27883997

Zickgraf HF, Ellis JM: Initial validation of the Nine Item Avoidant/Restrictive Food Intake disorder screen (NIAS): a measure of three restrictive eating patterns. Appetite 123:32–42, 2018 29208483

Zipfel S, Wild B, Groß G, et al: Focal psychodynamic therapy, cognitive behaviour therapy, and optimised treatment as usual in outpatients with anorexia nervosa (ANTOP study): randomised controlled trial. Lancet 383(9912):127–137, 2014 24131861

Ziser K, Rheindorf N, Keifenheim K, et al: Motivation-enhancing psychotherapy for inpatients with anorexia nervosa (MANNA): a randomized controlled pilot study. Front Psychiatry 12:632660, 2021 33597901

Disclosures

The Guideline Writing Group and Systematic Review Group reported the following disclosures during development and approval of this guideline:

Catherine Crone, M.D., is employed by the Inova Health Systems as Vice Chair of Education, Department of Psychiatry, George Washington University/Inova Consultation-Liaison Psychiatry Fellowship Program Director, and Director of the Psychiatry Consult Service at Inova Fairfax Hospital. She reports no conflicts of interest with her work on this guideline.

Laura J. Fochtmann, M.D., M.B.I., is employed as a distinguished service professor of psychiatry, pharmacological sciences, and biomedical informatics at Stony Brook University and deputy chief medical information officer for Stony Brook Medicine. She is a co-investigator on a grant funded by NIMH and has received payment for grant reviews for the NIMH. She consults for the American Psychiatric Association on the development of practice guidelines and has received travel funds to attend meetings related to these duties. She reports no conflicts of interest with her work on this guideline.

Evelyn Attia, M.D., is Professor of Psychiatry at Columbia University Irving Medical Center and Professor of Clinical Psychiatry at Weill Cornell Medical College. She directs the Center for Eating Disorders at New York-Presbyterian Hospital and the NYS Psychiatric Institute. She receives research funding from NIMH and royalty payments from UpToDate. She reports no conflict of interest with her work on this guideline.

Robert Boland, M.D., receives compensation for his work as a psychiatry director of the American Board of Psychiatry and Neurology, Inc. He is a consultant for MCG Health, where he participates in peer review of care guidelines; however, Dr. Boland is not involved in guideline development. He reports no conflicts of interest with his work on this guideline.

Thomas J. Craig, M.D., is retired and has no conflicts of interest with his work on this guideline.

Javier Escobar, M.D., is Associate Dean for Global Health and Professor of Psychiatry at Rutgers University-Robert Wood Johnson Medical School. He receives funds from NIMH, Fogarty-National Institute of Health, and University of California, Los Angeles for research collaborations. He reports no conflicts of interest with his work on this guideline.

Victor Fornari, M.D., M.S., is Professor of Psychiatry and Pediatrics at the Zucker School of Medicine and is employed by the Zucker Hillside Hospital of Northwell/Health. Dr. Fornari receives royalties from NOVA Publishing as well as grant funding from PCORI for his role in both the MOBILITY Trial and the START Trial. In addition, Dr. Fornari receives funding from the New York State Office of Mental Health for his work with Project TEACH. Dr. Fornari is the psychiatrist on a study funded by SAMHSA entitled STRYDD. He reports no conflicts of interest with his work on this guideline.

Neville Golden, M.D., is employed as the Marron and Mary Elizabeth Kendrick Professor of Pediatrics and Chief of the Division of Adolescent Medicine at Stanford University School of Medicine. He is a co-principal investigator on a grant funded by the NIH/NICHD. He reports no conflicts of interest with his work on this guideline.

Angela Guarda, M.D., is employed as an Associate Professor of Psychiatry and Behavioral Sciences at the Johns Hopkins School of Medicine and is Director of the Johns Hopkins Eating Disorders Program. She receives current grant funding and support from the Klarman Family Foundation and the Stephen and Jean Robinson Eating Disorders Professorship Fund. She reports no conflicts of interest with her work on this guideline.

Maga Jackson-Triche, M.D., M.S.H.S., is employed as the Department of Psychiatry Vice Chair for Adult Behavioral Health and as Vice President of Adult Behavioral Health Services, UCSF Health, at the University of California at San Francisco School of Medicine and Medical Center. She reports no conflicts of interest with her work on this guideline.

Laurie Manzo, M.Ed., R.D., L.D.N., CEDRD, is employed part time as a Senior Clinical Nutritionist at the Massachusetts General Hospital. She is also affiliated with the Eating Disorders Clinical and Research Program at Massachusetts General Hospital. She reports no conflicts of interest with her work on this guideline.

Margherita Mascolo, M.D., CEDS, is employed by Alsana: An Eating Recovery Community as their Chief Medical Officer. She is also an Assistant Professor of Medicine at the University of Colorado Health Sciences Center. She has no conflicts of interest with her work on this guideline.

Karen Pierce, M.D., is employed full time in private practice. She is an associate clinical professor at the Feinberg School of Medicine. Dr. Pierce receives travel funds from the American Academy of Child and Adolescent Psychiatry for her work on various committees: AACAP-PAC board, Co-chair of the Advocacy Committee, and member of the Collaborative and Integrated Care Committee. She has no conflicts of interest with her work on this guideline.

Megan Riddle, M.D., Ph.D., M.S., is a clinical instructor at the University of Washington and is employed at the Eating Recovery Center. She has no conflicts of interest with her work on the guidelines.

Andreea Seritan, M.D., is employed as a professor of psychiatry at the University of California, San Francisco (UCSF) School of Medicine and UCSF Weill Institute for Neurosciences. She receives grant support from NIMH. During work on this project, Dr. Seritan also received grant support from the Defense Advanced Research Projects Agency, the Parkinson's Foundation, and the Mount Zion Health Fund. She reports no conflict of interest with her work on this guideline.

Blair Uniacke, M.D., is an Assistant Professor of Clinical Psychiatry at Columbia University Irving Medical Center and the Unit Director of the New York State Psychiatric Institute's inpatient eating disorders unit. Her research is supported by the Brain and Behavior Research Foundation and Columbia University's Irving Institute for Clinical and Translational Research. She reports no conflicts of interest with her work on the guidelines.

Joel Yager, M.D., is employed as a Professor of Psychiatry by the Department of Psychiatry, University of Colorado School of Medicine. He receives honoraria for serving as a Section Editor for UpToDate. He also receives honoraria and travel expenses for occasional academic grand rounds and professional association presentations. He reports no conflicts of interest with his work on this guideline.

Nancy Zucker, Ph.D., is employed as Professor of Psychiatry and Behavioral Sciences at Duke University School of Medicine and as Professor of Psychology and Neuroscience at Duke University. She receives funding from the National Institute of Mental Health. She reports no conflicts of interest with her work on this guideline.

Individuals and Organizations That Submitted Comments

Erin C. Accurso, Ph.D.
Judith Banker, M.A., LLP, FAED
Jessica Barker, MPS
Timothy D. Brewerton, M.D., DLFAPA, FAED, DFAACAP
Douglas W. Bunnell, Ph.D., FAED, CEDS-S
Jennifer L. Carlson, M.D.
Theresa Carmichael, R.D.
Elijah Castle
Richard Chung, M.D., FAAP
Mary Ann Adler Cohen, M.D., FACLP, DLFAPA
Sarah Coles, M.D.
Zafra Cooper, D.Phil., B.A., D.Clin.Psych.
Scott Crow, M.D.
Riccardo Dalle Grave, M.D.
Kamryn T. Eddy, Ph.D.
Nancy Ellis-Ordway, Ph.D., LCSW
Rana Elmaghraby, M.D.
Lisa Erlanger, M.D.
Gemma D. Espejo
Ellen Fitzsimmons-Craft, Ph.D.
Guido K.W. Frank, M.D.
Melissa Freizinger, Ph.D.
Stein Frostad, M.D.
Cathryn A. Galanter, M.D.
Maalobeeka Gangopadhyay, M.D.
Stephanie Garayalde, M.D.
Josie Geller, Ph.D., R.Psych.
Marwan El Ghoch, M.D.
Deborah R. Glasofer, Ph.D.
Mark A. Goldstein, M.D.
Daniela Gómez, M.D., Ms.C., CEDS, FAED
Sasha Gorrell, Ph.D.
Raquel Halfond, Ph.D.
Michelle Haneberg, B.A.
Marcia Herrin, Ed.D., MPH, RDN, LD, FAED
Lisa Hutchison, M.D.
Leanna Isserlin, M.D., FRCPC
Karen Jennings Mathis, Ph.D.
Jillian G. (Croll) Lampert, Ph.D., R.D., L.D., M.P.H., FAED

Kerry L. Landry, M.D., M.S., CEDS-S, FAPA, DFAACAP
Finza Latif, M.D.
Janet Lee, M.D., FAAP
Daniel Le Grange, Ph.D., FAED
Diana C. Lemly, M.D.
Molyn Leszcz, M.D., FRCPC, CGP, DFAGPA
Jessica Luzier, Ph.D., ABPP, CEDS-S
Nasuh Malas, M.D., M.P.H.
Alison Manley, M.S., LPC
Laura A. Markley, M.D., FACLP, FAAP, FAPA
Margaret Metzger, B.A.
Lindsey Miller, Pharm.D., BCPP
Lisa B. Namerow, M.D., FAACAP
Anne Marie O'Melia, M.S., M.D.
Emma Palmer, Pharm.D., BCPS, BCPP
Rebecka Peebles, M.D.
Teresa Pigott, M.D.
Charles W. Portney, M.D., DLFAPA, FAED
Juana Poulisis, M.D.
Maria Rago, Ph.D.
Marcella M. Raimondo, Ph.D., M.P.H.
Mae Lynn Reyes-Rodríguez, Ph.D., FAED
Roxanne Rockwell, Ph.D.
Ellen S. Rome, M.D., M.P.H.
Stacey Rosenfeld, Ph.D.
Jeffrey D. Roth, M.D.
Emily Rubenstein, M.A., LMFT
Shiri Sadeh-Sharvit, Ph.D.
Patricia Santucci, M.D., FAPA, FAED
Janet Schebendach, Ph.D., R.D.
Mujeeb Shad, M.D.
Jennifer Shapiro, Ph.D.
John Shemo, M.D., DLFAPA
Jordan Shull, M.D.
Gabrielle Silver, M.D.
Allison Spotts-De Lazzer, M.A., MFT
Danielle Stutzman, Pharm.D., BCPP
Anna Tanner, M.D.
David L. Tobin, Ph.D.
Janet Treasure, Ph.D., FRCP, FRCPsych

Eva Maria Trujillo Chi Vacuan, M.D., FAED, CEDS, FIAEDP, FAAP
Susan Beckwitt Turkel, M.D., FACLP
Tracey Wade, BScHons, MClinPsych, Ph.D.
Stephenie Wallace, M.D., FAAP
B. Timothy Walsh, M.D.

Mark Warren, M.D., M.P.H.
Therese S. Waterhous, Ph.D., RDN, CEDRD-S
Fran Weiss, LCSW-R, BCD, DCSW, CGP
Christina, Wierenga, Ph.D.
Kathryn J. Zerbe, M.D.
Stephan Zipfel, M.D., Ph.D.

Academy for Eating Disorders
Academy of Consultation-Liaison Psychiatry
American Academy of Child and Adolescent Psychiatry, Physically Ill Child Committee
American Academy of Family Physicians
American Academy of Pediatrics
American College of Neuropsychopharmacology
American Group Psychotherapy Association
American Psychiatric Association Assembly Representative – Psychiatric Society of Virginia
American Psychiatric Association Council on Children, Adolescents, and Their Families
American Psychiatric Association Council on Consultation-Liaison Psychiatry
American Psychological Association
American Society of Clinical Psychopharmacology
ANAD-National Association of Anorexia Nervosa and Associated Disorders
Boston Children's Hospital
College of Psychiatric and Neurologic Pharmacists
Comenzar de Nuevo A.C./TecSalud
Eating Recovery Center
F.E.A.S.T
International Association of Eating Disorders Professionals
Mental Health America
Minnesota Psychiatric Society
REDC Consortium
Royal Australian and New Zealand College of Psychiatrists
Society for Adolescent Health and Medicine
Willamette Nutrition Source, LLC

Individuals That Participated in the Expert Survey

Erin C. Accurso, Ph.D.

Sarah E. Altman, Ph.D.

Ellen Astrachan-Fletcher, Ph.D., CEDS

Chase Bannister, M.D., M.S.W., LCSW, CEDS

Karen Beerbower, MS, RD, LD/N, CEDRD, FIAEDP

Kelly Bhatnagar, Ph.D.

Kathi Bjerg, RD, LD

Lindsay P. Bodell, Ph.D.

Cara Bohon, Ph.D.

Mary E. Bongiovi, M.D., Ph.D.

Harry A. Brandt, M.D.

Kathryn S. Brigham, M.D.

Timothy D. Brewerton, M.D., DFAPA, FAED, DFAACAP

Wayne A. Bowers, Ph.D.

Gayle E. Brooks, Ph.D.

Cynthia M. Bulik, Ph.D.

Douglas W. Bunnell, Ph.D., FAED, CEDS

Deb Burgard, Ph.D., FAED

Simona Calugi, Ph.D.

Jennifer L. Carlson, M.D.

Giuseppe Carrà, M.D., M.Sc., Ph.D.

Massimo Clerici, M.D., Ph.D.

Danielle Colborn, Ph.D.

Frances Connan, MRCPsych

Carolyn Costin, M.A., M.Ed., MFT, FAED, CEDS

Steven Crawford, M.D.

Scott J. Crow, M.D.

Antonios Dakanalis, M.D., Psy.D., Ph.D.

Riccardo Dalle Grave, M.D.

Jennifer Derenne, M.D.

Michael J. Devlin, M.D.

Julie Duffy Dillon, M.S., RD, NCC, CEDRD

Suzanne Dooley-Hash, M.D.

Angela Celio Doyle, Ph.D.

Kamryn Eddy, Ph.D.

Marci Evans, M.S., RDN, CEDRD

Angela Favaro, M.D., Ph.D.

Fernando Fernandez-Aranda, Ph.D., FAED

Martin Fisher, M.D.

Ellen E. Fitzsimmons-Craft, Ph.D.

Kelsie T. Forbush, Ph.D.

John P. Foreyt, Ph.D.

Sara F. Forman, M.D.

Victor Fornari, M.D., M.S.

Melissa Freizinger, Ph.D.

Donna M. Friedman, M.S., LPCI

Stein Frostad, M.D.

Jennifer L. Gaudiani, M.D., CEDS

Ata Ghaderi, Ph.D.

Marwan El Ghoch, M.D.

Daniel E. Gih, M.D., FAPA

Marci E. Gluck, Ph.D.

Andrea B. Goldschmidt, Ph.D.

Mark A. Goldstein M.D.

Janna S. Gordon-Elliott, M.D.

Leah L. Graves, RDN, LDN, CEDRD, FAED

Angela Guarda, M.D.

Nupur Gupta, M.D., M.P.H.

Elizabeth Hamlin, M.D.

Ann F. Haynos, Ph.D.

Beate Herpertz-Dahlmann, M.D.

Marcia Herrin, Ed.D., M.P.H., RDN, LD, FAED

Hans W. Hoek, M.D., Ph.D.

Leanna Isserlin, M.D., FRCPC

Joel Jahraus, M.D., FAED, CEDS

Vanderlinden Johan, Ph.D.

Craig Johnson, Ph.D., FAED

Rosalind Kaplan, M.D., FACP

Debra K. Katzman, M.D., FRCPC

Pamela K. Keel, Ph.D.

Kelly Klump, Ph.D.

Jillian G. Lampert, Ph.D., M.P.H., RD, FAED

Yael Latzer, D.Sc.

Maria C. La Via, M.D.

Daniel Le Grange, Ph.D.

Diana C. Lemly, M.D.

Christian R. Lemmon, Ph.D.

Ronald Liebman, M.D.

James Lock, M.D., Ph.D.
Katharine L. Loeb, Ph.D.
Carolina Lopez, Ph.D.
Jennifer D. Lundgren, Ph.D., FAED
Jessica Luzier, Ph.D.
Brad A. MacNeil, Ph.D., C.Psych
Marsha D. Marcus, Ph.D.
Laurel Mayer, M.D.
Michelle Lee Mayfield Jorgensen, M.D.
Carrie J. McAdams, M.D., Ph.D.
Liz Blocher McCabe, Ph.D., LCSW
Kim McCallum, M.D., CEDS, FAPA
Susan L. McElroy, M.D.
Philip S. Mehler, M.D., FACP, FAED
Rachel Millner, Psy.D., CEDS
Madhusmita Misra, M.D., M.P.H.
Lauren Muhlheim, Psy.D.
Stuart B. Murray, DClinPsych, Ph.D.
Rollyn M. Ornstein, M.D.
Carol B. Peterson, Ph.D.
Emily M. Pisetsky, Ph.D.
Charles W. Portney, M.D.
Marcella Raimondo, Ph.D., M.P.H.
Daniel Richter, M.D.
Renee Rienecke, Ph.D.
Giuseppe Riva, Ph.D.
Roxanne Rockwell, Ph.D.
Ellen S. Rome, M.D., M.P.H.
Shiri Sadeh-Sharvit, Ph.D.
Jessica K. Salwen, Ph.D.
Janet Schebendach, Ph.D., RD

Jessica Setnick, M.S., RD, CEDRD
Jennifer R. Shapiro, Ph.D.
Mima Simic, M.D., MRCPsych
April Smith, Ph.D.
Brad E.R. Smith, M.D.
Allison Spotts-De Lazzer, M.A., LMFT, LPCC, CEDS
Robyn Sysko, Ph.D.
Mary Tantillo, Ph.D., PMHCNS-BC, FAED
Jennifer J. Thomas, Ph.D.
C. Alix Timko, Ph.D.
David L. Tobin, Ph.D.
Stephen Touyz, BS c, Ph.D.
Janet Treasure, Ph.D., FRCPsych
Eva Trujillo, M.D., FAED, FIAEDP, CEDS
Mary Ellen Trunko, M.D.
Jessica VanHuysse, Ph.D.
Kristine Vazzano, Ph.D.
Tracey D. Wade, Ph.D.
Glenn Waller, D.Phil.
Mark J. Warren, M.D., M.P.H.
Therese S. Waterhous, Ph.D., RDN, CEDRD
Christina E. Wierenga, Ph.D.
Jennifer E. Wildes, Ph.D.
Denise Wilfley, Ph.D.
April N. Winslow, M.S., RDN, CEDRD
Lucene Wisniewski, Ph.D., FAED
Kathryn Zerbe, M.D.
Stephanie Zerwas, Ph.D.
Stephan Zipfel, M.D.